Get Off Your Path

...and get on the path to a

self-sustainable healthy lifestyle!

Written By

Dr. Jon Petrick

Dedication

To the most important person in my life, my amazing daughter "Gianna".

You are my "WHY"

-Daddy

To my special friends Mark Reese and Scott and James Ruggels.

You have helped me stay humble and honorable.

-D.J.P

Acknowledgments

I would like to thank Dr. James Adkins, whose mentoring, consistency of the message, and knowledge has been the impetus for not only delivering this book, but for having the courage to champion a revolution in healthcare.

A special thanks to my good friends and colleagues for sharing their knowledge and expertise: Dr. Joseph Pelino, Dr. P. Michael Leahy, Dr. Francis Murphy, Dr. Jim Kiernan, Dr. Lois Laynee, Mr. Grey Cook, Mr. Greg Rose Dr. Golan Nissim, Dr. Roy Nissim Dr. Michael Jarembek, Dr. Dale Buchberger, Dr. Thomas Alfreda Jr, Dr. Leo Germin, Tony and Kathryn Bonello, Dr. Joseph Huginin, Dr. Kintaro Oku, Dr. Chris Barney, Dr. Mike Crovetti, Kelly Eubanks, Stan Efferding and Marty Greenbaum. You are all true pioneers and creators of positivity, and you inspire greatness. Because of you, millions of people are living happier, healthier and more fulfilled lives.

Finally, I want to thank my amazing and supportive immediate family. The fact we are all so tight and close has always been the motivation for me to try new things. Thank you to my dear mother Nikki Wilkie, father Jack Petrick, Step-father James R. Wilkie (USMC) and siblings Jeff Petrick, Brooke Ross and James Wilkie, Jr. Thanks for always keeping it real.

Get Off Your Path

Rave Reviews

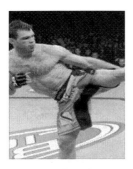

"I have taken some of the hardest hits and have had some of the craziest injuries you can think of and Dr. Petrick always has a way of putting me back together. He put me in the hyperbaric oxygen chamber, which helps with traumatic brain injuries, not that I had had any...ha ha... but it helps with recovery." **– Forrest Griffin – UFC Champion**

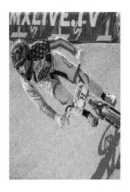

"Dr. P is the best! I have known Dr. P for a very long time, he knew me as a little boy when I was racing BMX around the west coast. When the results came and we found out that I would be representing our country in London, in the Olympics, in BMX, I am not sure who was more excited...me, my parents or Dr. Petrick." **– Connor Fields – USA Olympic Athlete**

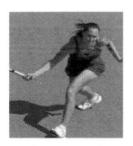

"I have had my fair share of nagging injuries. No matter what injury I showed up with, Dr. Petrick was willing and able to help me. I am grateful to have met him and to get treated by him. He is truly a great doctor." **– Jelana Jankovic – Professional Tennis**

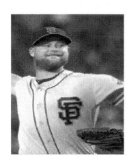

"I have been around the league and I have had the very best doctors in the world and I can honestly say that Dr. Petrick is one of the very best. He is not afraid to push the limits with treatment and care Sometimes you just need someone to just get it done and done right!" **– Chad Gaudin - MLB Pitcher**

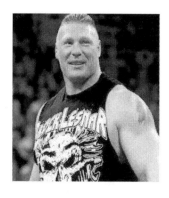

"Over the years, I have had my fair share of injuries. No matter if it was a recent injury or something that has been bothering me for a long time, Dr. Petrick helped me work through it. He helped me through some of the toughest times. He respects the athlete and work as hard as we do to keep at our best." – **Brock Lesnar, UFC and WWE champion**

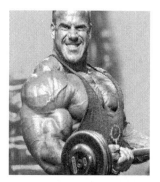

"I knew no matter what; if I was going to make it back to the top, I needed Dr. Petrick on my comeback team. I am really lucky because I can get the best care in the world, and trust me I do. I came to Dr. Petrick because I have been all over the world and I can honestly say he is the very best." – **Jay Cutler - 4 Time Mr. Olympia**

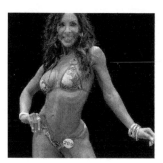

"Dr. Petrick and his magic hands keep my body functioning at the highest level. I am able to go all out during all of my workouts! I am so thankful to have met Dr. P, he is not only great at what he does but I also consider him a great friend!" - **Stacey Alexander - Professional Bikini athlete**

Table of Contents

Get Off Your Path

Introduction

A few years ago there was a Hollywood movie and sitcom called "Limitless." The plot of the movie and recent television show have a very unique and interesting perspective as the main character chose to take a special pill that would allow him limitless control over his entire brain. Can you imagine the amazing possibilities if you could turn on the trillions of neurons in your brain? And what if you had the ability to immediately decrease the stress that you were under by naturally producing nitric oxide in your body, decreasing your blood pressure and improving circulation of oxygen? Science has proven that adults can re-generate brain cells through diet, exercise, and a fundamental, self-sustaining lifestyle.

Here's a great example that shows the importance of being able to improve oxygen and nitric oxide in the body. Picture this...Kobe Bryant or Peyton Manning, in the last minute of the game, and they are called upon to lead their teams to victory. I bet they would want to have every single brain cell that they have turned on and ready to perform at the highest level.

Let's assume you were about to take a very important test, or preparing for a multi-million dollar business deal. The more brain cells that you have turned on, the more clarity, sharper and efficient your brain will work. If you had the power to turn it on, would you use it?

I was once asked by a group of friends and colleagues why I decided to write a book about **The Self-Sustainable Healthy Lifestyle**.

Well........ The answer to that question came slamming into me one day while I was riding in the car with my daughter. We had just left her soccer tournament where her team had lost 2-1 in the finals. Even though it was a close game, they lost nonetheless. My daughter plays

Goalie on her team, and I can promise you that the stress you feel as a parent, when it comes down to penalty kicks, is almost palpable.

Because I know my child very well, I could tell she was really upset about the loss. I told her "baby, it's ok, you did great…. losing isn't everything…….and losing is part of life……" AND I'll never forget her face when she turned to me with giant tears in her eyes, and she said, "Daddy, I hate to fail." BAMMM! I realized right then that I knew exactly what my daughter was feeling. Like my daughter, I hate to lose and I hate to fail.

See, for several years I had been trying hard to help all my patients become pain free and to perform at their very best, but when I took a long look back at the patients that I could not fix or help, they all had one thing in common: chronic pain caused in one way or another by inflammation and degeneration.

Due to either the foods they were eating, the way they were breathing, the amount of stress they were under, or the way their bodies moved, something was causing a lot of inflammation. The mucus caused by inflammation is the true root cause of almost all diseases. If I could teach my patients how to prevent inflammation, and to become knowledgeable and self-sustainable, I would be able to impact their lives permanently.

Inflammation is directly linked to obesity. It leads to degeneration in the joints, to faulty wiring in the brain and spinal cord, and is responsible for early aging and decay.

I thought to myself, "How can I stop failing, truly help these patients and affect their quality of life forever?" I wanted to address all of my patients' concerns under one roof. I wanted to change the way patients were being treated. I wanted to empower my patients, and enrich their lives by interesting them in a self-sustainable, healthy lifestyle.

So I sat down and using sound science, clinical experience and a lot of research, I developed a lifestyle program designed around decreasing inflammation, educating my patients on their bodies (inside and out) and interesting my patients in self-sustainable principles that they could apply immediately into their lives.

The program I now call the Self-Sustainable Healthy Lifestyle (SSHL) was originally created to teach patients how to increase oxygen to the brain, reduce stress through increasing the production of nitric oxide and to live healthier. I have now added a way to balance hormone levels, screen body movement patterns for asymmetries, determine which foods they're sensitive to and examine the DNA and the neurotransmitters to rule out any genetically linked issues that could eventually cause a disease.

The Self-Sustainable Healthy Lifestyle (SSHL) consists of three (3) key sets of protocols. The first set of protocols, which are the doctor applied, must be applied by a well-trained physician. The second consists of two groups of self-applied protocols designed to be performed at home. These protocols increase oxygen to the brain and increase nitric oxide production. The third is applying self-sustainable ideas like growing food at home, wind or solar alternatives, and other ways to become self-sustaining and to shrink the patient's footprint on the earth.

I have done the hard work and all the research, and I developed the SSHL program which is simple and easy to learn. If you apply the protocols discussed in this book, you will be able to increase the amount of oxygen being supplied to your brain and turn on the trillion brain cells begging for more O2. You will be able to use the self-applied movements, postures, stretches and exercises in this book on a daily basis to reduce stress and its effect on the body.

There are literally thousands of self-help books out there aimed to improve your overall potential or perceived success. However, most of them do not address the physical, mental or chemical stresses being placed on the body. Those books do not offer immediate ways to improve your life so you can live a happier, healthier, more fulfilled life.

This book is written for you to GET OFF the negative, unhealthy, sluggish path that you're on and start a path to a self-sustainable healthy lifestyle. You will immediately feel better than you have felt in a long time.

This Self-Sustainable Healthy Lifestyle book covers many easy to implement self-sustainable methods, protocols, processes and action steps such as: growing vegetables in your own home, getting the best night sleep possible, making sure you're exercising the right way for you. You will know how to live a truly self-sustainable, self-healing, self-sufficient, healthy lifestyle. All you have to do is **Get Off Your PATH**.

Dr. Jon Petrick

Chapter 1

Unforeseen Detours

Like many people, my life was on one path, and due to an unforeseen circumstance, it took a total detour and led me down a totally different path.

That detour, however, proved to be the best thing that could ever have happened to me. It forced me to make one of the biggest and best choices in my life, up to that time. That detour would forever positively change my life, even though I did not know it at the time.

Unfortunately, that unforeseen circumstance or detour in my life was a horrible automobile accident. While I was living in Phoenix, Arizona, I was on my way home one night from a Halloween party. And to make a long story short, the driver of the jeep I was in lost control and ran off the road. I was thrown violently from the jeep and ended up with major injuries.

I sustained serious injuries to my head, my neck, shoulder and the lumbar area of my spine. In addition to the pain, I had all the associated ever-so-wonderful neurological symptoms of numbness and tingling in my hands and feet. The pain was unreal, the sleeplessness and fatigue were unbearable, and being totally honest, I was really getting scared. There I was a young, healthy, in-shape guy, but at that moment I was in bad shape. My life was in a major downward spiral, and it was heading to the bottom fast. My job at the bank was now in jeopardy, my friendships were starting to feel strained, and I was becoming severely depressed.

I had gone to several different doctors, including many highly recommended chiropractic physicians, and nobody could help me. I was passed around from this doctor to this doctor. It seemed that none of them ever communicated, and I was just running around wasting time and money. I was told several times that I had permanent nerve damage, primarily on the right side of my body, to the extent that I couldn't even hold a glass of water.

Out of sheer coincidence, a coworker recommended that I see a physician by the name of Dr. James Adkins in downtown Phoenix. She said that she knew several people who Dr. Adkins had helped and they too had been told they had permanent conditions. Even though I was skeptical, out of sheer desperation I still went to the appointment.

I met with Dr. Adkins. He thoroughly explained to me in great detail the nature of my injuries and the consequences or probable outcomes. He gave me the hope I was desperately needing. He also explained that he was the only physician in Arizona, at that time, utilizing a technique called "Active Release Techniques."

Active Release Techniques (ART®) is a patented, state of the art, soft tissue, movement-based technique that treats problems with muscles, tendons, ligaments, fascia and nerves. ART was designed to free the adhesions that build up in the soft tissues after inflammation or injury has occurred. Unfortunately for me, the scars formed around the nerves and were causing a lot of pain and dysfunction.

I underwent several painful treatments, but I noticed an immediate and noticeable change after a very short time. In fact, the very first night after my first treatment was the first good night's sleep that I'd had in the months since the accident.

I continued treatment with Dr. Adkins for a few more months, and within a short period of time, he had fixed almost all of the nagging conditions and symptoms that I'd had. None of the other doctors, over the nine-month period since my accident, could even come close.

During my treatment I noticed that it was not just me. Every patient in his waiting room was reporting that they were feeling better (I heard the patients in his waiting room). When Dr. Atkins was able to help me and all those other patients, I knew right then I needed to make a drastic change in my life. One day during treatment the opportunity came to approach Dr. Adkins. I said to him: "I want to do what you do. Where do I need to go? How do I do it? And when can I start?"

He said they don't really teach Active Release Techniques outside of a chiropractic program. He said that I would first need to get my Bachelor's degree, and then I would need to obtain a chiropractic degree. That meant four years of medical school and that was after I received a Bachelor's Degree. So to say the least, there was a lot of schooling that I needed - a lot of distance between where I was at and where I wanted to be.

After his mentoring, I immediately enrolled in Cleveland Chiropractic College in Kansas City, Missouri. Within six months of first speaking to Dr. Adkins, I packed up my belongings in my small beat up car and was on my way to Missouri to attend Chiropractic College. My life's path changed the very moment I left Arizona and started school.

Even though Dr. Adkins said I would probably have to wait to take Active Release, by nature I am very impetuous and was not one to wait. As soon as I was accepted and enrolled in school I contacted Active Release headquarters in Colorado Springs. I asked if they could make an exception and allow me to take the course before I graduated from Chiropractic College. Luckily for me, they agreed to allow me to attend an upper extremity course. It was my first of many seminars while in chiropractic school, and my first certification was earned in Atlantic City, New Jersey, in 1995.

Even though Active Release was already around for about ten years, it was not widely recognized or well known. In fact, many people had never even heard of it, let alone practiced it. In 1995 I was the only one in my chiropractic college learning Active Release Techniques. It did not take me long to know that I was doing something pretty special. As I began to excel in our clinical or residency program, I noticed that I started to have a following. I was the intern with all the patients.

When I graduated in 1999, Active Release Techniques was the single most significant technique that allowed me to stand out in the crowd. ART gave me an automatic niche and drastically separated me from every other green-eared graduate coming out of Chiropractic College.

Where Do I Go Now

When I was deciding on where to set up practice, I had done a lot of research, and I had selected a few great locations. My final two cities that I settled on were Austin, Texas and Sacramento, California.

One day while visiting my parents in Las Vegas, Nevada, they were giving me a ride to the airport. My mom innocently asked me what I was looking for in a place to live and setting up my center. I had researched the answer for a long time and I told her, rather abruptly, I wanted to be around family, warm weather, and the opportunity to have a niche.

She said with a smile, "WOW! That sounds like you're describing Las Vegas." She was right. For whatever reason, I had never even once thought about Vegas. But when I sat down and really thought about it, it made total sense.

I would be the only physician certified in Active Release in the entire state of Nevada, which meant that I would have the immediate marketing advantage or niche that I was needing. Second, the weather in Las Vegas for nine months of the year is perfect. Third, I had immediate family living in Las Vegas and having their help would be crucial and paramount to success. Lastly, due to Las Vegas being such a vacation, seminar and convention mecca, with every airline and city having direct flights there, it was almost a no brainer... travel to and from Vegas would be easy. I thought that these qualities would be perfect for me to set up my center and that was that. I set my sights on Las Vegas, and in January of 2000 I moved to Las Vegas, Nevada.

They say that things happen for a reason. After my accident, I pretty well hit rock bottom - no money, a broken body and an uncertain future. But I was somehow led to Dr. Adkins, who not only became my saving grace, but the greatest mentor to shine some light on where I wanted to be in life, and I was now on a new path.

Little did I know, but Active Release Techniques wasn't going to be the only "out of the box" treatment or technique that I was going to learn and not the only path I would go down.

The "Jerry Maguire" Epiphany

I know that many of you may have seen the famous Tom Cruise movie "Jerry Maguire." The plot was based on the main character, Jerry Maguire (Tom Cruise), who was a successful sports agent with many high profile clients. After many years of making millions of dollars for his clients, he felt that the human element was now missing. He, in a sense, grew a conscience and realized that the most important thing in life was relationships. So he had a meltdown of sorts and wrote a paper (mission statement) for his colleagues to read. The paper he wrote was about caring more for clients, having less clients, offering them better customer service, really getting to know the clients, and building a strong honest bond. As I sat there watching the big screen movie, I had the same mental challenges. Then like in the movie, I had my very own epiphany.

5

After many years in practice, I was becoming frustrated at the lack of customer service, caring, compassion and understanding in healthcare. My patients were sharing horrible stories during their treatments with me. Some of their stories were downright disturbing, and they seemed to be a common trend in healthcare.

For the most part a patient's healthcare is dictated by whichever insurance coverage they own. They can only go to doctors who are on their insurance plan, whether they chose that plan or not and whether they liked the doctor or not. They had to simply take whatever care they were given and shut up and smile. Or, they could pay out of their pocket for care that their insurance should have covered in the first place.

I am not trying to beat up on an already broken system, but in all seriousness, our healthcare system is *literally killing* patients. It is estimated that over 400 patients per day die unnecessarily due to staff errors, wrong procedures, accidents, wrong prescriptions being administered, and "new" infections obtained inside our United States hospitals alone. This does not include the morbidity, mortality and suffering from millions of procedures that never were medically necessary in the first place.

I am not trying to be negative or pessimistic, but I am very concerned about healthcare and seeing it first-hand, I must do something about it. I have to make a stand and offer something different, something better. You're worth it! My patients are worth it!

So, even though I was finally running a very successful chiropractic business, I knew something was missing. I was searching for better ways to treat my patients. I wanted to offer the very best in patient care and customer service. I needed to find a solution as I was passionate about revolutionizing medicine. In my heart and from what my patients were sharing with me, I knew they were not getting great care, and often, patients were even being neglected.

I needed some help and guidance. I knew exactly where to go. I again reached out to my long time mentor and friend, Dr. James Adkins, and asked him for advice.

By this time Dr. Adkins's small chiropractic business that I once knew had grown from a tiny, one doctor operation into one of the largest multi-disciplinary spine centers in Arizona. I met with Dr. Adkins for several planning sessions and took his advice, which was to develop a unique but effective, multi-disciplinary treatment center specializing in customer care and blending allopathic and alternative medical practices.

I have included in this book, in my opinion, a few of the biggest challenges we are facing in healthcare today. It is these challenges that have led me to the self-sustainable lifestyle model— but keep reading, because in this book you will find optimistic, self-sustainable protocols that you can immediately implement to improve the quality of your life while taking control of your environment.

Correction needed number 1: Unnecessary Care
Simply put, there are way too many unnecessary and over-used procedures. This overuse accounts for almost one third to one-half of all of our health care costs in the United States. That means hundreds of billions of dollars are simply wasted. That is not including the half-a-trillion dollars wasted every year that can be attributed to lost productivity due to disability.

Correction needed number 2: Harm to Patients
As I stated earlier in this chapter, over 400 patients die every day un-necessarily due to errors, procedures, accidents, wrong prescriptions,

and "new" infections. Unfortunately, this issue is one of healthcare's ugliest and most common problems. The national statistics are nothing less than disturbing. Here's an example: it is estimated that 25% of Medicare patients admitted to the hospital will suffer some form of harm or mistreatment while staying in the hospital. Would you fly on a plane if you were told you had a one in four chance of landing safely at your destination? Probably not.

Correction needed number 3: Billions of Dollars are Being Wasted

A report by the Institute of Medicine Health suggests that at least a third to one half of all health costs are wasted or abused.

Correction needed number 4: Insensitive Customer Service or Care

I am constantly seeing and hearing about the horrible stories associated with the poor, disrespectful and un-empathetic care being delivered. Somehow administrators, nurses and doctors have forgotten that patients are people, too. Maybe they have forgotten that their patients are healthcare consumers. If patients were not bound to insurance carriers choosing their doctors, these bad doctors would never see a patient again if patients were not treated properly.

If patients were truly allowed to choose their own doctors, and better yet, interview their physicians first, and doctors had to compete for patients, you would see a dramatic change in the number of errors being made. You would also see a huge improvement in care and an increase in polite customer service. Those doctors who lack bedside manner, caring, compassion and love for their patients would starve.

Correction Number 5: Lack of Alternatives and Transparency

We have far more information available to us to purchase and select a new home or car than we do to choose where to go for health care. In this book and through my lectures, I provide my readers and patients with many easy, inexpensive and achievable alternatives to standard healthcare and ingenious ideas as to how to become self-sustainable.

The next step is for purchasers and consumers of healthcare to demand better: better treatment, better customer service and better communication from their insurance carriers, physicians and healthcare support staff. We need to keep the pressure on because that is the only way to encourage real change.

Although this was a very challenging, expensive and complicated endeavor, I decided to take Dr. Adkins' advice --- follow my heart and combine specialties. So, I restructured my entire business model and established the "New" Las Vegas Pain Relief Center, which is a multi-disciplinary pain center. My main objective is to be able to provide everything a patient would ever need. I want to revolutionize chiropractic, and medicine, and the way patients are being treated. I hope, with the help of some others, to usher in a new blended approach to healthcare.

Chapter 2

It All Starts With the Proper Intake and Interview

In order to properly treat someone, we need to know way more than just their age, weight and blood pressure. Our intake form and processes are loosely based on the Mackay 66 form written by Harvey Mackay. Harvey's golden rule is to really get to know your customer. We take pride in our level of patient care, and our goal is to establish a long-term, trusting relationship with each individual patient.

Although our initial interview form is comprehensive, here is an example of some of the few "Out of the Box" questions we ask our patients:

MEDICAL HISTORY (Current Condition of Health)_____

DOES CUSTOMER DRINK?_____IF YES, WHAT AND HOW MUCH?_____

IF NO, IS CUSTOMER OFFENDED BY OTHERS DRINKING?_____

DOES CUSTOMER SMOKE?_____IF NO, OBJECT TO OTHERS?_____

FAVORITE PLACES FOR LUNCH_____ DINNER_____

FAVORITE ITEMS ON MENU_____ _____

DOES CUSTOMER OBJECT TO HAVING ANYONE BUY HIS/HER MEAL?_____

HOBBIES AND RECREATIONAL INTERESTS_____

VACATION HABITS_____

SPECTATOR SPORTS INTEREST: SPORTS AND TEAMS_____

WHAT KIND OF CAR(S)_____

CONVERSATIONAL INTERESTS_____

WHOM DOES THE CUSTOMER SEEM ANXIOUS TO IMPRESS?_____

HOW DOES HE/SHE WANT TO BE SEEN BY THOSE PEOPLE?_____

It's important to ask all of these "out-of-the-box" questions, especially when we're working with high level professionals. We need to know what their likes or dislikes are, and then we can formulate a program based upon what the individual needs and wants. In other words, what makes them tick?

Once we have a clear understanding of who you are from your intake questionnaire and interview, we will then recommend the appropriate diagnostic work-up needed for you.

Some of the initial tests we use we'll talk about later in the book, like the Selective Function Movement Assessment, which we use to determine whether it's a mobility issue or a stability issue. Is it your joint(s) or your soft-tissue(s) affecting the joint? Once that's established, other exams come in to play as we continue to learn more and more about you and the issues keeping you from feeling great.

Based on the Functional Movement Screen (FMS), we'll design an exercise program around your lifestyle, your likes, dislikes and your hobbies or interests. If you're going to stand on the top of a "John boat" and fly fish for Tarpon, we'll train you on a "bosu" ball upside down and work on your balance and coordination.

Our patients' lifestyles need to be applicable to the treatment plan and the program we design. That's why the intake forms are so valuable. If you're an executive, we want to know information about the executive. I don't want to know his/her bank account. What I want to know is what he/she likes doing. What are his/her interests or hobbies? It's important to know these things because I can then structure the program based upon that information.

Once we get the food sensitivity test results, a diet applicable to what foods you like to eat vs. the foods you need to stay away from will be designed. That's the key. Not every meal plan or diet has to have a grueling aspect to it. What I mean is, instead of having a diet you won't follow or stay on because you don't like the foods, we suggest foods that you like, but change a few things around like portion control and show you healthier ways to cook. You're going to say: "That isn't so bad."

Not everyone's lifestyle needs are the same, so we design programs to suit every individual patient's lifestyle the best we can.

Chapter 3

"Out of the Box"

Your first appointment will be like a "meet and greet." It's a personal meeting where we can see if there's a connection and start to build trust. We'll ask questions to establish your motivation like: where you're at mentally, what your long term goals are, and how I can manage expectations. We determine whether you are ready to push your body as well as your mind. We'll talk about self-sustainability, being able to maintain it, and making your life simpler. Before we even start, we need to know what you do right, what you do wrong and what we need to work on and with. So, a good clinical evaluation is very important to be successful.

I ask different types of questions than most typical medical doctors or physicians because I want to attach to the patient's personal side. I really want to find the kid inside of each patient again, to help rid them of the 'Peter Pan' Syndrome. I'd love to coin that phrase, because that's the truth. It's like the Peter Pan story. When Peter stopped believing in FUN and became slow, lazy, and boring --- basically, Peter became an adult. People don't frolic and play anymore as adults. We don't skip, jump or swing from trees. We get caught up on all the material possessions and money.

Thankfully, there is some optimism, and we are now starting to see changes in the exercise paradigm. Adults are starting to act like kids again. Organizations and groups are holding events like Spartan Races, Tough Mudders, and now you see TV shows like the American Ninja Warrior. These events help encourage adults to get outside, to jump around, play in the dirt, and have some FUN.

How I rehabilitate my patients is based on sound science, but most

Importantly, we make it fun. We challenge our patients to get active and permanently correct the issues. By implanting our SSHL protocols that are youthful, we see more adults getting back to activities that they did as children. However, we still have this societal impact that says we can't do that and we should not act like a kid. It is that path that needs change.

After that first interview we have, we will find out so much good information about where we're going to be able to make changes in your life. It isn't just hearing your goals; it's allowing me to be able to formulate a program, to give you what you want/need and the right plan to actually achieve those goals.

Here's an example: What if you lived in Florida and said, "I want to fish the Keys." That's a whole different thing than if you said, "I'd like to run a marathon." You're going to need a totally different training program. If you're wanting to fish the Keys, then I have to provide proper exercises that will improve your stability. We would train on a balancing platform, so that when you're standing up there, ready to cast that rod, you're balanced and safe.

The interviews that I have with my patients are very important. There's a distinction between the intake paperwork and the intake interview. The interview is a must, and the key to secure success. Not every part of life has to have a grueling aspect to it, and the interview allows us to make sure it doesn't.

Our clients' lifestyles are applicable to the treatment plan and the program we put them on. That's why the intake forms are so valuable. Another example: If you are an executive, we want to know specific information about *you,* the executive. I don't want to know your bank account information. What I want to know is what you're doing on a daily basis. What type of executive are you? How high is your stress level? It's important to know that because I can structure your program based upon that information.

A Successful Mindset Requires Action

Inactivity = motionlessness, which means that you're stagnating, not moving forward in any aspect of your life. You know you need to make changes and that you have to put them into action, but you just don't, or can't, do it.

At some time in your life you, probably had someone tell you that you couldn't do something that was important to you. Either you're your worst enemy, or you just didn't have a great enough support system in your life. Whatever the case may be, if you don't believe in yourself, you won't be able to achieve your dreams and goals, whether they be in business, family or health. Those who struggle with self-esteem issues have a harder time with their success mindset.

You don't believe you are worthy, yet everyone else is. You believe you can't lose ten pounds. You don't believe that you can eat healthier. More important, you believe that you don't deserve to better yourself. Maybe in the back of your mind you think you deserve better, but your fear paralyzes you. You need to get out of your mindset, know that you can make positive changes, and plan for your success.

Even if your mind is screaming "you can't do it," you still need to try. Many people are tripped up by believing before they take action, as opposed to taking action first. By taking action first and seeing the results, you're better able to believe that you can accomplish what you set out to do. We are not measured by our successes we are measured by our efforts for trying.

Your self-confidence goes up a notch every time you complete or even attempt a task. Taking small steps up the ladder, not taking too many rungs at a time, helps your mindset to develop stronger. Remember, slow, steady, and the one who takes action, wins the race.

Those with a fixed mindset frequently evade taking any action because they are afraid to come out of their comfort zone. They know what's safe, they know they're good at it, so that's where they tend to stay. If they take a step and it doesn't work out, they feel like a failure, and won't ever try again.

Many will keep going because they have that fire in them, while some will never try again. Those with a fixed mindset need that action to free them up for the potential that is skulking deep inside them.

If you can't do the little things, you won't be able to do the big things

As funny as it may seem, making your bed may seem meaningless, but it could possibly be the first positive thing that we do that day. The wisdom of this simple act has been proven many times over and over.

I once watched Admiral McRaven address the University of Texas class of 2014. His speech was very moving to me because it emphasized the importance of the little things.

He said, "If you make your bed to perfection every morning, you will have accomplished the first task of the day. It will give you a small sense of pride and completion, and this will encourage you to complete another task and then another and then another; and by the end of the day, that one mundane task completed will have turned into many tasks completed. It also reinforces the fact that the little things in life matter, and if you can't do the little things right, then you won't be able to do the big things right. If by chance you have a miserable day, you will at least come home to a bed that you made. A made bed will give you the encouragement that life will be better tomorrow. So if you want to change the world, start by making your bed."

Define the Actions You Need to Take

Many people, who make all-encompassing statements about what they want their success to look like tend, to come up with over-the-top goals that are either too vague or totally out of their control.

One of my favorite examples of unclear goals is someone saying, "I want to make a million dollars." Or if someone says, "I want to lose 30 pounds." Those are good goals but they are too broad of statements. In order to be successful, you need to know the who, how, what, where and when actions that need to be taken in order to achieve your goal.

Your statements should be: "I want to make a million dollars in the next six months through my stock portfolio and this is the action needed," and "I want to lose 30 pounds in the next three months by exercising and eating healthier and this is the action needed." Your goals are now definable, planned out and organized; therefore, they are more attainable.

You are now able to focus on the stock market, on healthy recipes, on exercise techniques, on a fitness coach or a mentor. All of these steps move you toward what has been defined as your ultimate goal.

However, don't totally focus on where you will be someday. Focus on where you are at the moment, and take daily action towards your goals. Dan Gamble, USA Gold Medalist, once said: "What did we do right, what did we do wrong, and what do we need to work on." I ask this of myself every day, every week and every month to make sure I am being positive, productive and profitable.

When you were a baby, you didn't just stand up and walk. You had to crawl first, then you took baby steps to get to where you wanted to go. You had to put one foot in front of the other; otherwise, you would stumble and fall, but there was a process that took place. Once you got going you never stopped.

Achieving mini goals on a regular basis builds trust in the process and shows you that the world is wide open because you have a growth mindset. Mini goals are evidence of your consistent accomplishments, which reinforces your belief in yourself.

Action strengthens beliefs. People who have a fixed mindset will often avoid taking action. They want to do what they know is safe, what they're already good at. Because if they take an action step and it doesn't work out, it will make them feel as if they've failed. This is a hard thing for most people with a fixed mindset to experience.

Some will never take that leap of faith again, while others will keep going because they want it bad enough. It's action that takes someone with a fixed mindset and frees them up to the potential lurking inside of them.

The reason that you don't want to focus on only one broader single goal is because that it leads to a fixed mindset. You're in a constant state of failure until that goal is reached. If you're achieving mini goals on a regular basis, then suddenly the world is wide open to you because you have a growth mindset – you can see evidence of your consistent accomplishments and it reinforces your belief in yourself.

7 Habits That Lead to a Strong Successful Mindset

To get what you want, whether it's in your personal or professional life, you have to learn to do what works. For most people, this means creating a habit. But a habit isn't something that never changes. A success habit is always evolving.

Habit #1 - Make sure what you want is really what you want. Don't do something just because you *think you should.* Check in with yourself every 30 days to make sure that the path you're on is the one you want to stay on. Doing this prevents you from ending up with business models that don't satisfy you.

Make sure you're not abandoning something out of fear of failure. There's a big difference between doing what's right for you and doing something that feels easier.

I suggest making a one year, two year, five year and a ten year plan of attack for every area of your life. **YOU MUST WRITE IT DOWN** and check it monthly to ensure that you are strictly following your plan. I use mine as a measuring stick and compass to make sure I am on par.

Habit #2 - Begin every day with motivation. These are things that work to get you to take the next step. For example, if you need to go for a run to clear your head and get some time to think, then do that. If you need to use specific habits every morning in order to get into the flow, then let those habits be what compel you to get into your day.

Starting off with motivational reminders is like eating breakfast in the morning – it helps fuel you throughout your day. You also want to spend a minute or two looking back over your day and being proud of what you did accomplish.

While I was in Chiropractic College, I needed constant reinforcement that I could do it. As a constant reminder for me to push and work harder and longer, I hung motivational signs that I made around my apartment. A few of my favorite motivational signs were:

- "Your enemy is up already."
- "Leaders are like eagles, they don't flock - you find them one at a time."
- "Attitudes are contagious. Is yours worth catching?"
- "If you can't out read them, then out work them."
- "Anger is the wind that blows away all reason."
- "In a 100 years it won't matter how big your bank account was,

or what type of car that you drove, but what will matter is the affect you had on the life of a child."

Habit #3 - Don't chase success to the point that you stop dreaming. Your success begins with an idea, a hope, a dream. If you go all out, driving hard, keeping your nose to the grindstone, you can reach the point where your mindset becomes fixed.

All you can see is the end result rather than the journey. Remember that on your way to getting what you define as success, you will never have these days filled with learning curves again.

Sometimes it becomes a chore to just blast through a task list – especially if you forget about why you're doing everything. If your goal is to live on the beach in a nice home, make sure you routinely revisit those plans to keep you inspired with your action taking.

Habit #4 - Make sure you leave room to grow. You need to have a success mindset that keeps you learning even when you feel you've made it. There's always something else that you can learn. Seek out new resources online, books, new niche leaders who teach things from a different perspective – anything that helps round out your education.

Habit #5 - Answer to someone else. You want to have someone in your life that you're accountable to. Make time to meet with someone who can help keep you on track for reaching your success. You want this person to be someone who can tell you when you're driving yourself too hard and someone who can help steer you around pitfalls.

Sometimes you won't have a specific person in your life capable of doing that. You can turn to a paid life coach or even join a forum of like-minded, positive individuals all striving for their own success.

Habit #6 - Learn to trust yourself. When you go after what you want in life, there will always be someone waiting to tell you that something is either a good idea or a bad idea. Everyone has a built-in alarm that will sound if something is off. Trust your Gut Feelings.

You'll feel it as knots in the pit of your stomach or as a sense of unease. When you begin trusting yourself in these situations, it helps you develop a sense of self-confidence and strength.

Habit #7 - Understand that roadblocks are going to happen. You have to determine ahead of time that you won't give up - you won't surrender a growth mindset to a fixed one. Roadblocks can often be used as character builders.

They can strengthen your resolve and help you learn to become more resourceful as you find another way to do what you want to get done. If you become too comfortable with your efforts, you often don't achieve the ultimate success that you're after.

Having a strong mindset in life, whether for your personal or professional satisfaction, requires a combination of positive thoughts and verifiable action steps.

Whenever you do something that you start to feel a bit of shame over (like quitting on a project), ask yourself if you're doing it because you don't believe enough in yourself to succeed.

If that ends up being the case, take the task and break it up into micro-sized mini goals that you can work on to see if you're capable of making progress that way. Sometimes, it's the simple fact that a project seems too big that ruins many of the best plans.

It's also a good idea to surround yourself with action-taking, positive people. Take inventory of the kinds of people you're currently surrounded with. Do they always complain about everything?

Do you find yourself commiserating with people stuck in the same boat as you? If so, jump out and swim to shore because that boat is sinking fast, and you don't want to be swallowed up by the pity party they're throwing for themselves.

Seek out motivational experts whose thoughts align with what you find inspiring. Tune in to their messages or read their books daily as if you're taking a vitamin designed to prevent illness.

Over time, you're going to become someone others look to for support, and you'll notice they come to you with fixed mindsets. They'll be attracted to the positivity you project. Make sure you turn their mind around, rather than letting their limited thoughts infect you.

Chapter 4

The Anatomy of a Chiropractor

Chiropractic – Which Means "To do or perform by Hand"

The world of chiropractic care is truly fascinating. We are routinely asked a variety of questions about chiropractic care and what we actually do in our office. In response to all the fantastic questions, I decided to put together this short chapter to get your questions answered.

Why is Chiropractic Care so Popular?

Well, for one, it is effective. A recent survey conducted by Consumer Reports found that over sixty-five percent of all people who seek chiropractic care for pain report experiencing "a lot" of relief from their symptoms.

Another reason chiropractic care continues to gather favor from the masses is that it is a safe, natural, and non-invasive way to treat health ailments. That means that your chiropractor will treat your condition without prescribing you medications, putting you through surgery, or causing you any further damage. Chiropractic philosophy involves a holistic, whole body approach to treating problems. Therefore, you know that when you go to a chiropractor, you will receive care that is centered on providing your entire body what it needs to get better, without asking more of your body.

May people also gravitate toward chiropractic care because it can be easily integrated into whatever healthcare plan they already have in place. Chiropractors work closely with other doctors, specialists, therapists, nutritionists and other healthcare practitioners toward your wellness goals. Even if you currently see a doctor for your health issue, chiropractic care can be a worthwhile addition.

What Does a Chiropractor Do?

A chiropractor is trained to use a well-rounded approach to caring for your health ailment. That means your treatment plan will be multifaceted. It is likely to be comprised of any combination of treatments, including spinal manipulation. This is the cornerstone of chiropractic care, and no matter what other treatments you receive, you will receive spinal manipulation during every session with a chiropractor. The process is exactly what it sounds like: your chiropractor will manipulate your spine in order to achieve optimal vertebral alignment, and thus counter the negative symptoms you are experiencing.

The Basics of Spinal Manipulation

Once you have your first appointment over with and out of the way, your chiropractor will formulate a treatment plan that will best suit your needs. One integral part of this treatment plan will be a process called spinal manipulation. The frequency and duration of spinal manipulation sessions you receive will be determined by your condition, as well as your body's response to chiropractic care. Here is what you should know about spinal manipulation:

The goal of spinal manipulation. The chiropractor's goal is to align the vertebrae of the spine to their optimal position. What is optimal positioning of the vertebrae? Ideally, the vertebrae should sit uniformly on top of one another, allowing plenty of space in-between each disc for the proper functioning of the nerves. Therefore, the purpose of the spinal manipulation process is to correct vertebral misalignments (also called subluxations).

Techniques used during spinal manipulation. A spinal manipulation is done by way of a series of manual techniques, as performed by your chiropractor. Each chiropractor has a unique way of doing things and uses different techniques for different patients, depending on their individual circumstances. As such, if you ask one hundred different patients what a spinal manipulation involves, you might get one hundred different answers. The one unifying factor of all spinal manipulation techniques is that they involve the application of pressure to one or more areas of the spine, with the intent of budging the vertebrae out of the wrong position and into the right one.

How spinal manipulation works to alleviate symptoms. Herniated and bulging discs, as well as swelling of the surrounding tissue, can place a lot of pressure on the nerves between the discs. These nerves must communicate with the rest of the nervous system, and their functioning is severely stunted by this pressure. As previously mentioned, when the vertebrae of the spine are properly aligned, it allows as much space as possible between the discs. This, in turn, alleviates that detrimental pressure on the nerves, freeing them up to heal and once again communicate effectively with the rest of the nervous system. Damaged nerves send signals of distress – or, pain signals. Healthy nerves send messages of health and healing. Therefore, an aligned spine can work wonders for a multitude of health ailments.

What to expect during a spinal manipulation. You may or may not experience immediate relief from your first spinal manipulation. That is because your body is responsible for appropriately aligning itself (with the chiropractor's urging, of course), and the body is a creature (so to speak) of habit. It is not unusual for the spine to slip back into its previous, undesirable position after the first adjustment, simply because that is what it is used to. So be prepared that it may take more than one adjustment to feel immediate and/or lasting relief. It is also important to note that you can expect to experience some soreness or discomfort right after your alignment. This is perfectly natural, and will go away in very little time. Your body just needs to learn its new place and get comfortable in it.

Chapter 5

The Physician Applied Protocols

In this chapter I would like to touch on some of the successful **Physician-Applied** treatments and procedures that we offer in our center. It is critical that we first fix or correct the issues prior to teaching the self-applied protocols. All of these **Physician-Applied-Protocols** are discussed and supervised by a trained professional, and you should consult a physician before ever starting any physical fitness or diet program. Remember... there is power in knowledge.

Functional Movement Systems

When people ask me how I became successful or so knowledgeable in my skill set, the only truly real answer that comes to my mind is ... LUCK. I am simply lucky. I was lucky to have had so many amazing mentors in my life. It seemed that whenever I was ready for growth, I would reach out to the universe and a mentor would appear. I often had to be keen and smart enough to identify them, but they always showed up to guide me to the next level. I fully credit them and I am grateful for my mentors. They have dramatically impacted the way I practice, the way I physically train, and so many other areas of my life. My philosophies and corresponding set of tools used in practice are based on sound science, years of innovation, and current research and are utilized in almost all professional organizations.

In order for me to accurately diagnosis the true cause or source of a person's condition, I needed a consistent, accurate, reproducible, and dependable diagnostic process. When I first started my practice, there was no systematic tool to identify movement asymmetries or major limitations in functional movement patterns. What was out there was not reliable and was often way too difficult for a patient to understand. As my success started to grow and I started working with hundreds of professional athletes, I realized that it was a whole new level and I couldn't afford to be inaccurate. My methods had to work and my programs had to make sense.

So, I was searching for a process or set of protocols to rehabilitate my patients at the highest level. By pure luck I met Grey Cook, who was the developer of the Functional Movement Systems. I was immediately amazed at how easy he explained movement issues and how I, as a patient being screened, could actually see my own movement asymmetries and improve them.

Because the Functional Movement Systems are so accurate, we use it to promote a collaborative effort between our treatment, performance and rehabilitation professionals. The system is made up of two (2) main tools - *the Selective Functional Movement Assessment™ and the Functional Movement Screen™.* Both of these tools evaluate movement but are separated by a very clear distinct marker. That marker is pain. If movement produces pain, the individual would be sent through SFMA. If pain is not present, then the FMS is the appropriate tool. This systematic process allows clinicians to clearly match their intervention to the main problem of the patient. This model efficiently integrates the concepts of altered motor control, the neurodevelopmental perspective, and regional interdependence into musculoskeletal practice.

The Selective Functional Movement Assessment (SFMA)
The Selective Functional Movement Assessment (SFMA) is the movement-based diagnostic system designed to clinically assess seven (7) fundamental movement patterns in those with known musculoskeletal pain. The assessment provides an efficient method to systematically find the cause of symptoms, not just the source, by logically breaking down dysfunctional patterns and diagnosing their root cause as either a mobility problem or a stability/motor control

problem. The final diagnosis from the assessment is either (1) Tissue Extensibility Disorder (TED), (2) Joint Mobility Disorder (JMD) or (3) Combination of both.

Why the Selective Functional Movement Assessment?

Movement Matters - Movement quality is an essential component to reducing the risk of injury and reaching optimal levels of performance.

Systematic Approach - A reliable baseline to screen and evaluate movement is key to providing actionable and effective steps for performance and recovery.

Communication - The system allows for performance and rehabilitation professionals to speak the same language when communicating client progress and treatment.

Professional Network - Build a referral network for your business by connecting and collaborating with professionals who share your passion for functional movement.

The Functional Movement Screen (FMS®)

The Functional Movement Screen (FMS®) is the product of some of the most forward thinking minds in the physical medicine industry. Grey Cook, a friend of mine, developed and created the Functional Movement Screen which is a part of the Functional Movement System. The functional application of the screen and the practicality of the FMS progressions makes the training a perfect match for every individual patient.

Simplifying Movement

Simply put, the FMS is a ranking and grading system that documents and scores a patient's movement patterns that are essential to normal function. By screening these specific patterns, the FMS readily identifies functional limitations and the asymmetries that are the true cause of movement disorders, pain and degeneration. Functional Movement Screen (FMS®) consists of seven (7) full-body movement patterns that are critical to normal function. Each movement pattern is scored from 0-3, and a total score of 21 is the highest score a person can obtain. However, I must warn you… I have only had one or two patients who scored a 21 on their first time screened. The Ideal score is 14 or above. The research has determined that a patient is 8-10% more likely to have a disc injury in their neck or low back if their score is not 14 or better. The screen is excellent at picking out the small micro-movements asymmetries that are subconsciously affecting gait, posture and overall health.

I estimate that 80% of the patients that I treat, not including the ones with acute injuries, have major asymmetries that either were misdiagnosed or not diagnosed at all. Many of these asymmetries would have led to a replacement surgery if we did not identify the movement asymmetries early in the process. These asymmetries reduce the effects of proper functional training, limit physical conditioning, and distort the body awareness and performance.

This scoring system is directly linked to the most beneficial corrective exercises to restore mechanically sound movement patterns. Simply put, you can't afford to guess anymore. Your life is way too important.

My team of exercise professionals, trainers and practitioners monitor the FMS score to track improvement and to identify the most effective exercise program to restore proper movement and build strength in each individual. My patients come in all different shapes and sizes, so I must have a successful way to find, correct and prevent asymmetries in movement.

FMS Widespread Benefits

The FMS simplifies the concept of movement and its impact on the body. Its streamlined system has benefits for everyone involved - individuals, weekend warriors, exercise professionals, and all kinds of physicians. The FMS is being used by, or has been used by, the NFL, NHL, UFC, MLB, NBA, PGA and PBA, along with other organizations like Special Forces branches of the United States Armed Forces.

- Communication - The FMS utilizes simple language, making it easy for individuals, exercise professionals, and physicians to communicate clearly about progress and treatment. The more our patients understand the program, the more likely they are going to adhere to it.
- Evaluation - The screen effortlessly identifies asymmetries and limitations, diminishing the need for extensive testing and analysis. The most important thing is that the patients themselves notice and feel the asymmetries. When they actually see how these limitations are effecting them, they want to make a change.
- Standardization - The FMS creates a functional baseline to mark progress and provides a means to measure performance. Part of the science aspect where everything we do is consistent for quality.
- Safety - The FMS quickly identifies dangerous movement patterns so that they can be addressed and patients can avoid them immediately. It also indicates an individual's readiness to perform the specific exercises, so realistic goals can be set and achieved.
- Corrective Strategies - The FMS can be applied at any fitness level, simplifying corrective strategies of a wide array of movement issues. It identifies specific exercises based on individual FMS scores to instantly create customized treatment

plans. We have a plan for every patient.

The Active Release Techniques Soft-Tissue Management System

This technique I am obviously biased about as I feel it literally saved my life. Active Release was the technique used by Dr. Adkins to restore my body to full function after my accident. He was taught the ART protocols by Dr. P. Michael Leahy himself. Dr. Leahy is the creator/founder of Champion Health Associates and the respected inventor of Active Release Techniques®.

Dr. Leahy has been one of the Team Physicians for the Denver Broncos for more than 12 years. Dr. Leahy discovered and published the Law of Repetitive Motion and the Cumulative Injury Cycle, which has helped redefine prevention and treatment of work-related injuries.

What is Active Release Techniques?

ART treats conditions related to the build-up of adhesions and scar tissue in muscles, tendons, and ligaments. These adhesions cause several problems: muscles become shorter and weaker, the motion of muscles and joints are altered, and nerves can become compressed. As a result, the affected tissues suffer from pain, decreased blood supply, and poor mobility. ART claims to fix these issues by releasing trapped nerves and restoring the smooth movement of muscle fibers.

In an ART treatment, the provider uses his or her hands to evaluate the texture, tightness and mobility of the soft tissue. Using hand pressure, the practitioner works to remove or break up the fibrous adhesions, with stretching motions generally in the direction of venous and lymphatic flow, although the opposite direction may occasionally be used.

In the first three levels of the ART treatment, as with other soft-tissue treatment forms, movement of the patient's tissue is always done by the practitioner.

Every Active Release Technique (ART®) session is actually a combination of examination and treatment. The ART provider uses his or her hands to evaluate the texture, tightness and movement of muscles, fascia, tendons, ligaments and nerves. Abnormal tissues are treated by combining precisely directed tension with very specific patient movements.

These treatment protocols (over 500 specific moves) are unique to ART and allow providers to identify and correct the specific problems that are affecting each individual patient.

Why Active Release Techniques?

I am always asked the question: "Why is ART different?" Simply put, it is all in the motion. ART requires the patient to actively move the affected tissue in prescribed ways while the practitioner applies a specific tension, translation, and slight compression. Because the signals to the brain for movement (*Mechanoreception*) are faster than the signals to the brain for pain (**Nociception),** and the two signals can't occupy the same space and time; the pain signal, which is slower, gets there after the movement signal which lessens the pain response. The movement helps block out the pain.

ART is the gold standard in treatment for headaches, back pain, carpal tunnel syndrome, shin splints, shoulder pain, sciatica, plantar fasciitis, knee problems, and tennis elbow. These are just a few of the many conditions that can be resolved quickly and permanently with ART®.

Moreover, these conditions all have one important thing in common; they are often a result of overused muscles, tendons and ligaments. ART® stretches, separates, and releases soft tissue adhesions, and restores vascular and lymph circulation, increasing range of motion and strength. Sports injuries, whether at the professional level or in the backyard, cause significant pain, disability and loss of enjoyment of activities. Regardless of age, when injuries to bones, joints, muscles and ligaments occur, scar tissue develops. Scar tissue alters the normal biomechanics of the injured joint and causes the body to deposit unwanted calcium that results in the formation of bony spurs and arthritis.

Early and aggressive care is the best way to combat these unwanted tissue changes. Our multidisciplinary team's approach to injuries is second to none. Each treatment plan is unique and specific to each patient's specific injuries and is designed to promote a rapid and full recovery.

ARE YOU TWISTED?

The Twist is exactly what it sounds like—the physical and mental effects of continuous, unreleased stress over time. Whether physical, mental, or a combination of both, these stressors can, over time, cause or worsen chronic pain.

Physically, The Twist refers to an overall tightening of the right side of the body, with a corresponding lengthening on the left—often as a response to unmanaged mental or emotional stress. This "twisting" sets off a chain reaction, dragging nerves, blood vessels, ligaments, muscles, and bones out of place.

Chiropractic and other types of manual therapy often focus on "realigning" the parts of the body that have moved out of place—but without targeting the root stressors, The Twist will continue to reoccur. The SRM addresses the imbalances in Mental (stress), Physical (exercise to reduce the Stress), and Chemical (eating to reduce the Stress) health. These imbalances lead to a predictable Pattern we call the Twist. The pattern of the "Twist" is predictable and always shortened on the right side of the body, or twisted to the right. The right side of the twist is the contracted side; the left is the adaptive side.

If the "Twist" is not attended to or left untreated, it will lead to subluxations (partially displaced vertebra), muscle, tendon, ligament and facial dysfunctions. The dysfunction may not elicit pain; in fact, the twist that doesn't produce pain is worse and will often show up later in the disease process as a disc herniation, pinched nerves, meniscus tears, plantar fasciitis, and many more.

The Stress Relief Method – Physician Applied Protocols

The Stress Relief Method (SRM) is a unique nitric oxide releasing technique for prevention and treatment of stress-induced afflictions in the musculoskeletal, vascular and nervous systems. SRM utilizes two sets of patent-pending moves (1) Physician-applied protocols and (2) Self-applied protocols. They reduce tightness and prevent or resolve any restrictions associated with stress or fatigue. The SRM platform begins with a diagnosis of a *stress-induced constant tightness on the right side of the spine and body* known simply as "The Twist." We use three quick movement tests to determine the level of The Twist. The scale is 1-3, 3 being the most severe twist and 1 being mildly twisted.

The SRM targets the cranial, cervical, thoracic, lumbar, and sacral spinal nerves. My patients report experiencing instant stress and pain relief resulting in long-lasting effects felt for days/weeks, depending on the individual and the amount of stress they live in.

The SRM is designed to stimulate the Amygdala or limbic system in the brain which causes a release of nitric oxide, triggering parasympathetic muscle relaxation and increased blood flow throughout the body.

The nitric oxide blast, via the SRM, can provide a euphoric feeling and help sustain homeostasis in the cardio-pulmonary vasculature and the subsequent Neuro-musculoskeletal system (muscles, nerves, tendons, and ligaments). The movements work with your body's natural internal processes, rather than trying to control symptoms through external means only. The SRM can help achieve and maintain a healthy balance mentally, chemically, and physically. You will also read about the SRM self-applied movements in a later chapter. The self-applied moves are way more affective once the physician has released "Twist" first.

SRM creator/founder Dr. James E. Kiernan has published two separate studies regarding the role of increased levels of nitric oxide released during the SRM Physician-Applied treatments. Problems arise when individuals cannot produce nitric oxide, which occurs after years of stress. Stress forces nitric oxide producing segments of the mid-brain (amygdala) to atrophy or shrink. You can always tell when people can't produce nitric oxide, as they will try to talk through the entire treatment. The ability to disengage the mind from the chatter and relax has been lost. This is why the SRM self-applied program is so important. At home you practice the 12 SRM moves with the hope that the relaxed mind returns, and you will produce more nitric oxide.

Functional Internal Medicine

Functional Internal Medicine is a patient-centered model where we utilize diagnostics, interventions, and treatments that heal our patients. We aim to treat mind, body and soul. Instead of treating symptoms, we focus on the entire individual to improve and cure their ailments.

Dr. Andrew T. Still, M.D., instilled basic tenants in all of his students, which are still expressed in today's new generation of students. His four basic philosophies include: structure and function, the unity of function, the body's ability to heal itself, and the artery reigns supreme.

 A closer look shows us that when our structure is corrupted, the function is diminished. A simple example is when a patient breaks or dislocates a bone. When the body changes its physical form, functionally, the body has to change, too. Conversely, when our body encounters functional changes, we change the body's form. We see this in patients with diabetes and the development of diabetic peripheral neuropathy. The unity of function shows us that our body works as whole unit, like a masterpiece of precision. When we suffer disease or injury, this puts stresses on the rest of our systems, appreciates the infectious process which snowballs into sepsis and then multi-system organ failure, where our body works to regain hemostasis and heal ourselves. This is best accomplished when we have adequate blood and lymphatic flow so they are able to perform their specific functions.

Why are hormones so important?

Hormones are critical to our body's chemistry. They carry messages throughout our body, and they affect everything from growth to sexual development to our daily moods. Our bodies rely on hormones to function properly. When a hormonal imbalance occurs, it triggers symptoms that affect our health in various ways. Most of the time our hormones become unbalanced due to age, but this is not the only reason. There are other factors that can affect a person's hormone levels. Hypogonadism is a disease in which the body is not able to produce normal amounts of testosterone due to a problem with the testicles or with the pituitary gland that controls the testicles.

These symptoms can also be caused by various underlying factors including thyroid problems, diabetes, and depression. A blood test is the best way to diagnose a low testosterone level. A medical condition that leads to an unusual decline in testosterone may be a reason to take supplemental testosterone. Our male patients receive a blood test that tests for 11 areas of deficiencies, 17 for women. A comprehensive physical exam is completed for all patients. Once the results of a patient's blood test are reviewed by the physician, they will decide if a patient needs their hormones balanced or not and the best course of treatment.

Testosterone is a hormone primarily produced in the male testicles. A few benefits of testosterone for men is that it promotes a healthy sex drive, increases strength and muscle mass, bone density, red blood cell production, and sperm production. As men grow older, their testosterone levels gradually decline. This happens to all men, not just a few. Women also need testosterone, even though they need lower doses than men. It enhances mood, energy levels, sex drive, and ensures bodily functions flow smoothly.

Testosterone replacement therapy can improve the signs and symptoms of low testosterone in men by getting testosterone to optimal levels. Patients have less chance of struggling with these symptoms when their testosterone levels are balanced. If levels are low, patients experience reduced sexual desire, insomnia or other sleep disturbances, increased body fat, reduced strength, depression, have trouble concentrating or memory loss.

We recommend losing fat and increasing muscle mass through a personal training program to accomplish your personal goals. Balancing hormones is only one aspect of ensuring our patients lead a healthy life. Their personal fitness and nutritional intake are also extremely important. They must be managed specifically to each patient's needs and supervised by a physician. My colleagues Dr. Thomas Alfreda, Jr. and Professor Tony Bonello are the Co-Founders of

Health4life 'Age Management Medicine' headquarters in Las Vegas, Nevada, and they handle the functional medicine portion of our self-sustainable healthy lifestyle.

Injection Medicine

In my opinion injection medicine, although beneficial, really does not fix anything, but more specifically is used to manage pain and inflammation in the area being administered. We use it only as an adjunction to our standard physical medicine therapies to solely relieve inflammation. When you have an inflamed joint, we order an injection to the area which is usually a low grade steroid or anti-inflammatory to minimize the swelling and decrease sensitivity in the area. I'll give you an example: If a nerve root is swollen and inflamed and it's pressing against the disc, it's going to cause a neurological symptom very similar to what would be considered a disc herniation or a nerve root entrapment. However, if the nerve root receives an injection of a corticosteroid, it will lessen the inflammation and decrease the swelling of the nerve, hence decreasing the pain. Healing doesn't take place until the inflammation is relieved.

The problem with injections or steroids is that they are only a temporary fix and have been known to cause additional damage and disruption of the tissue matrix. There's typically an underlying biomechanical issue that is causing the nerve to swell. The corticosteroid injection is by no means an end-all for treatment. It is just an adjunct to our program for special circumstances.

Orthopedic Relationships and the Self-Sustainable Healthy Lifestyle

Surgeons, Sports Medicine Physicians and Physiologists usually have a great understanding about orthopedic treatments and the type of care we provide. Many Orthopedic physicians refer to our self-sustainable protocols because the pre-habilitation methods that we utilize aid them with their patient's recovery outcomes. When a patient goes through a proper pre-habilitation program prior to any surgical procedure, the outcomes are dramatically improved. Research has proven that conditioning, prior to an operation, returns patients to their normal daily activities 60% faster than those patients that had no pre-op conditioning or pre-habilitation. The combination of a great surgeon and a skilled ART, SRM, FMS doctor is incredible.

One of my favorite orthopedic physicians that I work with is my friend and colleague Dr. Michael Crovetti, D.O. His philosophy is treat the injury, train the injury, and, if that doesn't work, bring it back to him and he will repair the injury. His vast knowledge of rehabilitation and pre-habilitation makes him what I would call an "out of the box surgeon." Dr. Crovetti understands that surgery is the last resort and recommends every non-surgical attempt to prevent a procedure through rehabilitation and training. But in the end, when surgery is the only option, with his skilled approach, his patients are ready for action days after surgery.

Non-Surgical Spinal Decompression

Many times the damage is too great, but you seek to avoid surgery at any cost. You often need a non-surgical approach. For the severe cases of spinal degeneration, nerve root impingement, and disc herniations, we use Non-Surgical Spinal Decompression, which is a non-invasive treatment for acute and chronic spinal pain associated with stenosis, herniated, ruptured, bulging or degenerative discs. It is safe and effective without the normal risks associated with invasive procedures such as injections, anesthesia or spinal surgery.

Spinal decompression works through a series of 15 one-minute alternating decompressions (using a logarithmic decompression curve) and relaxation cycles with a total treatment time of approximately 30 minutes. During the decompression phase, the pressure in the disc is reduced and a vacuum type of affect is produced on the disc. This increases the *Nucleus Pulposis's* (inner nucleolus of the disc) ability to use oxygen and nutrition. The decompression or traction causes the oxygen and nutrition to be diffused into the disc allowing the *Annulus*

Fibrosis (the outside hard cartilaginous tissues) to heal.

Hyperbaric Chamber

America is experiencing an epidemic of sports-related concussions, leading to at least mild-moderate permanent brain injuries. These kinds of brain injuries do not heal by themselves, and the brain damage from concussions only gets worse with repetition and time. Most of these injuries occur during practice and often go undiagnosed.

The impacts of these hidden *in-the-brain* injuries can include short- and/or long-term memory loss including difficulties with verbal communication, decreased motor skills, deviations from normal behavior and drug addiction (which is often a form of "self-medication" to quiet the over-activity in the injured brain). Insomnia and dementia are two of the most common complaints.

Fortunately, there is finally a break-through medical solution, a high-pressure, pure oxygen therapy known as hyperbaric oxygen therapy that repairs the brain insults caused by concussions. This new technology-based treatment has just been adopted by many professional organizations and teams, like the San Diego Chargers, to help their players. Dozens of other current and retired players from across the National Football league are using hyperbaric oxygen therapy to heal their brains and to either prevent or recover from "post-concussive syndrome," which – in extreme cases – can cause dementia and early death.

This may be new "news" to most Americans, but the serious impact of concussions among veterans is much more widely known. What's not widely realized until lately is that a brain injury – whether from the blast of a roadside bomb or a helmet-butting tackle – cause the same kind of long-term, debilitating brain injury. However, Dr. Ann McKee, a Boston University School of Medicine researcher who conducted a study for the Veteran's Administration, recently told CNN that "we found the same damage to the brain in veterans as we did with pro-athletes."

Worse, traumatic brain injury – TBI – contributes to horrific suicide rates among America's veterans and has been linked to several suicides in the NFL. An average of 22 Afghan and Iraq veterans take their lives every day – while hundreds of thousands of other vets suffer each day from the awful, debilitating effects of Post-Traumatic Stress Disorder, PTSD.

Fortunately, what these veterans are experiencing is becoming more widely understood. Researchers and medical experts are beginning to search for answers and ways to treat these individuals. However, what's not well known or understood is that each year similar kinds of traumatic brain injuries happen to millions of civilians as well, and this happens without nearby explosions or concussive forces. Worse, these kinds of injuries are not making the news, so little is being done to prevent them or treat them. Each year more than four million Americans face this problem, including hundreds of thousands of school-aged kids playing contact sports or just "being kids." What this means is that this kind of life-threatening injury is far more common than most people realize.

For instance, an auto accident as slow as nine miles per hour can cause a mild to moderate traumatic brain injury, or TBI. A simple fall can trigger a TBI with long standing implications. However, perhaps the most common cause of a brain-related injury involves participation in a contact sport.

The statistics are frightening. According to a recent report about sports concussions that was issued by the (CDC) Centers for Disease Control and Prevention:

- 3,800,000 sports-related concussions were reported in 2012. This is double the number of concussions reported in 2002.
- Thirty-three percent (33%) of all sports concussions happen at practice.
- Thirty-nine percent (39%) is the amount by which cumulative concussions are shown to increase catastrophic head injury leading to permanent neurologic disability.
- Forty-seven percent (47%) of all reported sports concussions occur during high school football.
- One in five high school athletes will sustain at least one sports concussion during their season.
- Thirty-three percent (33%) of high school athletes, who experience a sports concussion, report two or more concussions during the same year.
- Including concussions not reported through the health system, four to five million sports-related concussions occur annually, with rising numbers among middle school athletes.
- Surprisingly, 90% of most diagnosed concussions do not involve a loss of consciousness.
- An estimated 5.3 million Americans live with a traumatic brain injury-related disability.

The worst-case scenario for damage caused by repeated concussive injuries is known as Chronic Traumatic Encephalopathy (CTE), a debilitating and potentially fatal, long-term condition which is caused by repeated blows to the head. These cumulative blows damage brain tissue and lead to the build-up of an abnormal protein in the brain. These kinds of repetitive concussive injuries put thousands of professional and amateur athletes at risk of coming down with this chronic degenerative brain disease.

CTE has recently been linked to many deaths of pro football players including:

Tom McHale, who played for the Tampa Bay Buccaneers, Dave Duerson, a starter for the Chicago Bears, and Junior Sau from the San Diego Chargers. In a limited study at Boston University's CTE Center, researchers analyzed the brains of former NFL pros. They found nearly 60 former pro football players suffered from CTE, which can only be diagnosed after someone has died.

And of course, every boxing fan knows of the current and sad condition of the one-time world heavyweight champion Muhammad Ali. Ali's reduced mental capacity is a highly visible public tragedy, but it is representative of the hidden, life-long suffering experienced by thousands of current or former professional athletes.

For over a decade, I have been a part of the medical team on Fox Sports' Ultimate Fight Championship reality television show. In addition, I've worked as a medical professional with the Toronto Blue Jays minor league program, the Las Vegas '51s, and many members of other professional sports teams and organizations. This experience has given me an up-close and personal understanding of how repetitive head injuries – even fairly mild ones – can begin to effect individuals' abilities to operate at peak mental efficiency. Throughout the years, I have looked for ways to ease or reverse the brain damage athletes, veterans and traumatic brain patients suffered.

The solution I've found is hyperbaric oxygen therapy.

This HBOT therapy involves immersing an individual in pure oxygen at 1.5 to 2.5 times normal atmospheric air pressure for 60 minutes, infusing their blood – and all the body's cells – with pure oxygen.

Oxygen stimulates healing and optimum performance at the cellular level. It is great for healing injuries and the after-effects of surgery, but it is also the only solution I could find for healing concussion-caused TBIs. It's not just the red blood cells that are filled with oxygen, but also every cell in the body, including the plasma.

Sports stars, like Joe Namath, have experienced remarkable brain-function and life-quality improvements using hyperbaric oxygen. In fact, Namath was so impressed with his improvement that he has invested $10 million dollars into hyperbaric treatment research to document what he already found in his own life – that, for athletes, hyperbaric oxygen therapy can be a game-changer.

This has a tremendous implication for professional athletes – football, hockey, soccer, UFC and other contact sports players – as well as for amateur athletes, victims of falls and/or car accidents. Regular HBOT treatments also help other non-brain injuries heal much faster, but HBOT treatment prevents head injuries from becoming TBIs. "Sugar" Shane Mosely uses the HBOT treatment immediately after a fight to prevent a TBI. For those who've experienced a TBI-causing concussion, the benefits are important. It is a simple relationship - brain function equals quality of life – which are both restored from HBOT.

The process at the Hyperbaric Institute of Nevada in Henderson (perhaps the most state-of-the-art HBOT treatment facility in the Las Vegas Valley) is second to none. Our standard procedures go something like this:

1. Individuals (after a very thorough medical work-up) are usually

referred from their treating physician, such as myself. Working with a doctor who understands the positive benefits of HBOT will help ensure a more comprehensive treatment – and recovery. Our initial brain injury workups include the use of a Functional Movement Screen, which looks for pattern deficiencies or abnormal movement patterns that can be linked to brain trauma.

2. Then the individual is given a special kind of brain scan which is called a "qualitative EEG" or qEEG, using advanced computer technology. This sophisticated, "base-line" scan provides a real-time 3D video of the brain in action, showing if, where, and how severely the brain has been injured. It also provides a means of measuring progress during recovery, the "before" of a "before-and-after" medical evaluation.

3. When the brain is injured, the body has a hard time properly regulating hormone production, so we recommend specific blood tests or blood panels to establish appropriate baselines or the amount of injury.

4. Then all of our patients, who we suspect of breathing issues, go through "airway restoration training" or breathing coaching. When a patient suffers a head injury, the body loses its ability to sequence normal breathing patterns, and we must reteach the body how to breathe again. That process, and the protocols we teach, make certain that there is no interruption in the normal breathing sequences, and we can maximize oxygen to the brain.

5. I advise all of my professional athletes, especially my MMA fighters, to have a baseline brain scan. It is my estimate that at least 80 percent of them actually have some kind of hidden traumatic brain injury. Most of them have had injuries during practice or sparing. I have heard horrific stories of fighters not even remembering their way home after practice.

Short-term recommendation: They should have four to five dives *before* each fight, and from eight to twelve dives *after* a fight – more if there's been an obvious head-blow or they were knocked unconscious and fewer if there was no apparent concussive injury.

Long-term recommendation: For that 90 percent who show evidence of long-standing TBI, I prescribe a course of 60-80 one-hour HBOT treatments at 1.5–2.5 times atmospheric pressure, with intermittent brain scans after 25-30 and 50-60 dives.

My recommendations also apply to all athletes who participate in all contact sports – football, hockey, soccer, lacrosse, basketball and baseball.

Chapter 6

Self-Applied Protocols

Group One: Oxygen – A Breath of Fresh Air

In this chapter I will share some of the most important and successful SELF-APPLIED treatments and procedures that we teach in our center. Because the self-applied protocols are so important, I have decided to give them, and the people who developed the techniques, their own chapter. The self-applied protocols are proven to improve oxygen uptake and increase nitric oxide production. They are to be implemented after you have completed a thorough examination and treatment from a trained professional.

We have all heard that you can't learn Karate from a book. It is also virtually impossible to implement the right protocols at the right time without instruction. But the great news is that once you're properly taught the self-applied protocols, you will never forget them. You'll be able to change your body's chemistry, mood and manner whenever you want or need to. You will be able to reduce the amount of damage that chemical, mental and physical stress plays on your body. You will need to have a trained SRM and airway restoration coach teach you the protocols first.

Laynee Restorative Breathing patterns are designed for daily home usage. We have to teach you how to sequence your breathing properly first before we send you home to breathe and bobble. Fortunately, how fast you improve all depends on you. How committed are you to turning on those trillions of neurons in your brain?

We use heart rate variability, CO_2 levels, mouth pieces, and a few other breathing tools to make sure we are making the correct and positive changes. The information we collect is used to monitor progression and set up baselines for oxygen saturation. We will restore stability to the airway with proper sequencing. The neurological sequencing associated with proper breathing and decreasing stress keeps inflammation down to a minimum.

It is absolutely critical that you, as a patient, buy into your own health and that takes 100 percent control, while accepting full accountability for improvement. We require frequent progression checks and home projects designed around improving the oxygen delivery to your brain.

We teach the self-applied protocols and procedures and provide ongoing care, diet, and exercise expertise. Whether it's more energy, healing faster after surgery, increased strength, more patience, better sex or a better restful night's sleep, the missing ingredient is Oxygen saturation and Nitric Oxide production.

Let's be honest... the first thing you think of when you think about oxygen is you think of breathing in and out, in and out. Don't worry, you're not alone; that is the first thing most people think when I discuss oxygen. However, the bad part is that most people do not breathe correctly, and it is playing a horrible toll on their bodies and their life. There is a reason it is called the respiratory SYSTEM, and it is not just the lungs and/or the nose, which is just the first portion of the respiratory system. There is a perfect sequence or cascade of neurological, chemical or electrical events that have to take place in order for proper breathing to occur and it starts in the NOSE. If you could take one thing away from this book, and it would be worth the price of admission, it would be TO BREATHE ONLY THROUGH YOUR NOSE.

Mouth Breathing is probably one of the most detrimental things we can do to our bodies. Our bodies are designed for special functions and your mouth is to eat and communicate; your nose is to breathe.

Ten Detriments from Mouth Breathing

1. Decreases oxygen availability in every cell
2. Stresses the immune system
3. Increases cortisol
4. No filtration system compared to the nose
5. Allows viruses direct access into the body
6. Increases mucus production
7. Decreases nitric oxide production
8. Increases blood pressure
9. Decreases ability of detoxification
10. Causes obesity

With the increased burning of fossil fuels, higher levels of smog, seasonal allergies and environmental lung diseases, increasing oxygen any way you can is a smart idea. If you are finding it difficult to breathe, try improving your oxygen levels by using the LOIS method 2-3 times per day and following the SRM self-applied, simple ideas in this book to improve your breathing.

How Your Body Uses Oxygen

Cellular respiration is a process through which the body releases energy stored as glucose, which is a compound composed of carbon, hydrogen and oxygen molecules. That energy is used to produce adenosine triphosphate, or ATP, which scientists call the "energy currency" of the cell. During respiration, the body oxidizes glucose and energy is released. The oxygen in the compound is reduced to water, while the carbon atoms in the glucose are released as carbon dioxide.

The Respiratory System

Scientists estimate that a human being breathes about 20,000 times a day, thanks to the components of the respiratory system -- the nose, throat, windpipe, voice box and lungs. The air that people breathe consists of several gases, with oxygen most important for cell growth and energy.

Carbon dioxide (CO_2), a waste gas, is produced when carbon is mixed with oxygen during cellular metabolism. Think of CO_2 as a liberator of oxygen. The higher the CO_2 levels, the more oxygen into the cell. It is possible, though, to have too much or too little carbon dioxide in the blood. Too much carbon dioxide can be associated with such conditions as Cushing's syndrome, Conn's syndrome, severe vomiting, restriction of blood flow, and lung ailments. Too little carbon dioxide, often caused by hyperventilation, can make muscles tense and cause people to become tense, anxious, stressed and **even aggressive.**

Oxygen keeps the cells alive and active. The more oxygen your brain gets, the more neurons get turned on; ergo, you will think clearer and sharper. We now know adults can grow new neurons.

How do you get oxygen into your body?

Oxygen, along with nitrogen and other inert gases, is found in the air around you. When you take a breath, air goes in through your nose and mouth, preferably your nose. The air passes through your trachea, or windpipe, and into airways called bronchi, located in your lungs. The airways branch off into smaller and smaller openings. At the end of the openings are alveoli, or tiny air sacs. The air bounces around in these tiny air sacs. Blood cells, in the very small blood vessels around these air sacs, pick up oxygen and carry's it throughout the body.

These very small blood vessels are called capillaries. Capillaries connect your arteries and veins. They are found all over the entire body. It is these small blood vessel capillaries in your lungs where oxygen is transported into your blood. This oxygen-rich blood then goes back into the left side of your heart where it gets pumped out to all parts of your body through your arteries. Then the blood and waste products, like carbon dioxide, return through your veins to the right side of the heart.

Throughout the rest of your body, these small blood vessels or capillaries carry the oxygen which is dropped off to your cells, and waste products, like carbon dioxide are picked up.

When the returning blood gets back to your heart, there is little oxygen left, but there is a larger amount of waste products. The blood goes into the right side of your heart and then gets pumped back into your lungs. The waste gases, like carbon dioxide, are passed from the blood through the capillaries into the air sacs. They are then breathed out through your lungs while more oxygen is being picked up by your blood cells. This air exchange happens quickly and often.

There is a chemical in your blood called hemoglobin which picks up and carries the oxygen in the blood. When there is oxygen, the hemoglobin turns bright red in color. As the oxygen levels decline, the hemoglobin turns a darker blue or purple in color.

What happens when the brain is injured?

When a part of the brain is injured, the brain cells become stunned and fail to operate properly, and subsequently, there is an interruption in the normal breathing sequences. These cells don't necessarily die, but they can no longer transmit the signals properly needed to signal the need for more oxygen. As a result, a section of the brain functions improperly – and over time, this "brain insult" gets worse and worse.

However, when the body's airway is taught to sequence properly and in severe cases immersed in high pressure pure oxygen, the stunned brain cells "wake up." They start demanding more oxygen, and the body starts to produce more Adenosine Triphosphate (ATP) which is energy. Because of the increase in oxygen and energy, new capillaries begin to grow, delivering more oxygen to the dying cells, and over a series of treatments, normal brain function is restored.

Restoring Proper Breathing Sequences

The Laynee Restorative Breathing Method™ explained

Breathing is the very first functional movement we ever develop as humans. Breathing is essential to our metabolic system, brain function, and our motor control system. When trying to coach someone to move better for flexibility, weight loss, strength, pre-habilitation, or rehabilitation, proper breathing instruction is paramount to a successful outcome. When you are thinking of functional training and how your programs are going, what is more functional than breathing! Breathing is something that you don't have to think about; you can't hear it and you barely notice it. It's easy, it's effortless, and it is so efficient that it gives you nothing but pure energy. Incredibly, most people do not know how to breathe or breathe wrong, and this has a huge negative impact on their lives. Sadly, they don't even know it until it's too late. We provide personalized breathing instructions to our patients and offer individual and group seminars aimed at helping fitness professionals incorporate effective, restorative breathing techniques into their lives and practices.

This breathing technique, or method, was developed by Dr. Lois Laynee "to generate a natural pure energy source to help the patient have a healthier and more fulfilled life, regardless of your age or gender." Although Dr. Laynee is based out of Phoenix, Arizona, she has taught at various colleges around the country, including the prestigious Yale College. She has been a true friend and inspiration for me, and her work will someday help revolutionize how we treat new moms and babies. I have been privileged to work with her on a very personal and special pioneering project. Her work could possibly change the world for children with Downs Syndrome by lessening the gene expression associated with the chromosomal defect for a narrow or an obstructed airways and the interruption of the cranial nerves.

The protocols that we teach restore the Autonomic Diaphragmatic breathing patterns that we all should have ingrained into our very make up. You must be able to have autonomic breathing patterns in order to have optimal recovery, performance, and life! We teach our patients to harness the one trillion neuron-connections, giving them ultimate mental clarity and focus, tweaking the human potential.

The Laynee Restorative Breathing Method™ consists of 4 very basic movements that ignite natural breathing from within. The following protocols are the first set of self-applied patterns you must learn. However, it is virtually impossible to learn them affectively without proper instruction and demonstration.

Dr. Laynee's Self-Applied Restorative Breathing Method™

1) LOIS breathing
    a. **"L"** Lips together
    b. **"O"** O shape with lips
        i. Tongue on roof of mouth
        ii. Teeth lightly closed - not clinched
    c. **"I"** Inhale and exhale through nose only
    d. **"S"** Silent slow breathing with soft swallowing
2) Bobble
    a. Inhale-Toes up- chin up
    b. Exhale-Toes down- chin to neutral (eyes open)
3) Pelvic Tilt
    a. Inhale-Anterior pelvic tilt
    b. Exhale-Posterior pelvic tilt

4) Cross Patterns

    a. Inhale-hand to head

    b. Exhale-opposite hand to opposite knee (Right hand to left knee)

    c. Swallow and hum

We use the Laynee Restorative Breathing Method™ to develop a road map to teach our patients to properly breathe and reap the benefits that proper breathing brings to every individual's health. Participants in one of our seminars will be able to effectively implement the Laynee Restorative Breathing Method™ in conjunction with SRM Self-applied and corrective exercise strategies for immediate improved function.

We teach proper breathing protocols, through the diaphragm, that ultimately completely changes their ability to heal, their ability to sleep, their ability to rest, and their ability to function.

The Laynee Restorative Breathing Method is an ideal 15-minute self-applied series of breathing protocols for *athletes, busy professionals, and aging adults*. We teach the Laynee Restorative Breathing Method so our patients can implement the protocols into their daily routine to enjoy a healthier, happier and a more fulfilled life.

Five simple things to do to improve your breathing

Open your windows. Nothing helps you breathe easier than getting fresh air. It's important to monitor your air quality! If you live in a particularly busy area that has a lot of smog, consider investing in an air filtration system and change your filters regularly.

1. **Grow a garden.** Think back to middle school when you learned about photosynthesis. If you remember, plants are basically inverse humans; they take in carbon dioxide and create oxygen.

This means by adding foliage to your home, you can increase the available oxygen.

2. **Get some exercise.** Give yourself a respiratory workout. As your breathing rate and depth increases, your lungs absorb more oxygen, and yes, that means more oxygen-rich blood tracing through your body.

3. **Drink more H2O.** Water is made of oxygen, so increasing your water consumption can increase the amount of oxygen in your blood. Start chugging.

4. **Yoga.** Begin a daily meditation or yoga routine that emphasizes deep breathing. Even if you just spend five to ten minutes sitting down and doing just the SRM or LOIS method, you can improve your oxygen intake and lower your stress levels.

5. **Diet.** Your diet can seriously impact oxygen levels. Certain foods can help improve your oxygen levels in the blood naturally. You should target iron-rich foods such as meats, poultry, fish, legumes and green leafy vegetables to improve iron uptake, which in turn improves blood oxygen levels. Stock up on green vegetables, like kale, broccoli and celery, in order to boost your oxygen levels and hopefully breathe easier. To kick-start your exciting new diet, we are going to create some amazing dishes and share our experiences with you! We suggest many healthy recipes that can help you improve your oxygen consumption. Use the techniques and protocols in this book to improve the oxygen levels of your blood. Most of these tactics will not only improve your health, but also improve your quality of life.

Chapter 7

Self-Applied Protocols

Group Two -Nitric Oxide

"The most important molecule in the human body... we can reverse cardiovascular damage with Nitric Oxide."
Dr. Louis J. Ignarro, Nobel Prize Laureate

Nitric Oxide - Your Body's Natural Stress Defense

Nitric Oxide (NO) is a chemical naturally produced by nearly every living cell in the human body – and plays a critical role in stress relief and immune response. Medical researchers and practitioners continue to explore its powerful health benefits. As a "signaling molecule," nitric oxide helps regulate blood flow, heart health, and cellular activity. Nitric oxide is now regarded as the most significant molecule in the body, absolutely crucial, thus leading to an overall sense of well-being. We use nitric oxide as a bio-marker that can be measured in saliva, blood and exhaled air. What we know from studies is that stress (chemical, physical or mental) reduces nitric oxide in the body. This causes early aging and increased buildup of lactic acid, which causes fatigue, decrease in range of motion, and an increase in pain. A reduction of nitric oxide is accompanied by vasoconstriction, or decreased blood flow, to all areas of the body, especially areas with the most pain. Less blood equals less oxygen, and we already discussed the effects of an un-oxygenated body.

Without sufficient nitric oxide, we can feel fatigued and worn down. It has the ability to expand blood vessels for better blood flow, which means more oxygen can reach the brain, heart, and other important organs. You can go the supplement route, or you can just boost nitric oxide production in the body naturally.

The soft tissue fatigue and restriction ultimately means a poor oxygen delivery system to all of the cells in the body. The Stress Relief Method (SRM) reduces or even eliminates the pain and stress so you can go about your daily activities with a reenergized feeling, both mentally and physically. You will have less frequent doctor visits and less paid medication dependency by implementing the protocols in this book.

If you have an existing heart condition or abnormal blood pressure, you should consult your healthcare professional before taking supplements to increase nitric oxide levels.

What is Nitric Oxide and How Does It Work?

Some people think nitric oxide is just a gas that makes us laugh at the dentist office, or it is a fuel racecars use to increase speed. But it is neither. Nitric oxide is a molecule that our body produces to help its 50 trillion cells communicate with each other by transmitting chemical signals throughout the body.

Nitric oxide has been shown to be important in the following cellular activities:

- Improves memory and behavior by improving the transmission of information between nerve cells located in the brain
- Improves the immune system to fight off bacteria and defend against tumors
- Regulates blood pressure by dilating arteries
- Reduces inflammation in the body
- Improves the quality of sleep
- Increases your recognition of sense (i.e. vision and smell)
- Increases endurance and strength
- Assists in gastric motility

Nitric Oxide and Heart Disease

There are thousands upon thousands of studies done on nitric oxide.

In fact the 1998 Nobel Prize for Medicine was given to three (3) scientists, who discovered the important role of nitric oxide and cardiovascular disease. That is where nitric oxide has gotten the most attention due to its cardiovascular benefits.

Even Alfred Nobel, the founder of the Nobel Prize, was prescribed nitroglycerin over 100 years ago to help with his heart problems. He was skeptical, knowing nitroglycerin was used in dynamite, but this molecule improved his heart condition. What he did not know was that nitroglycerin acts by releasing nitric oxide which effects blood vessels, increasing oxygen and blood flow.

The interior surface (endothelium) of arteries produce nitric oxide, and nitric oxide prevents the plaque from forming on the walls. When plaque builds up in your arteries, called atherosclerosis, which reduces the ability to produce nitric oxide, this is a Maytag of events that gets worse over time, which is why physicians prescribe nitroglycerin for heart and stroke patients.

Nitric Oxide and Erectile Dysfunction

Viagra, Cialis and other impotence medications work on the oxygen and nitric oxide pathways. One cause of impotence is unhealthy and aged arteries that feed blood to the sexual organs. The sexual organs fail to get proper blood and oxygen so obvious dysfunction occurs. Viagra, and the like, work by influencing enzymes in the nitric oxide pathway. This causes a cascade of enzymatic reactions that enhance nitric oxide production, which causes more blood flow and improved erections.

How to increase nitric oxide in your body

In this book, I explain the benefits of being able to increase the nitric oxide's production in your body naturally and effectively. The physician-applied protocols that I perform in my office, as well as the self-applied protocols that I teach, will increase your nitric oxide production. The most effective way to increase nitric oxide is to implement a specific set of exercises, postures, and patterns, and to improve your diet.

When you're actively running, doing cross fit, or working out in your boot camp, your muscles require more oxygen. As the heart pumps with more pressure to supply the demand requirement for more oxygen, the lining in your arteries and soft-tissues releases nitric oxide into the blood, which relaxes and widens the vessel walls, allowing for even more blood and more oxygen to enter the cells.

As we age, our blood vessels and nitric oxide system become less efficient due to free radical damage, inactivity, and poor diet. This broken system causes your veins and arteries to deteriorate and become leaky, and fall apart. Athletes and younger patients have the most optimal nitric oxide systems, reflecting their energy and resilience to the chemical, physical and emotional stresses being placed on their bodies. The more active the patient, the healthier they will feel.

Another way to increase nitric oxide is through diet, most notably by consuming the amino acids, specifically L-arginine and L-citrulline. Arginine can be found in nuts, fruits, meats and dairy, and directly creates nitric oxide inside the cells. The enzymes convert arginine to citrulline, and need to function optimally for efficient nitric oxide production.

We can protect those enzymes and nitric oxide by consuming healthy foods and antioxidants, like fruit, garlic, vitamins C and E, Co-Q10, and alpha lipoic acid, thus, also allowing you to produce more nitric oxide.

Nitric Oxide for Athletes and Bodybuilders. Increasing nitric oxide has become the new secret weapon for athletes and bodybuilders. Athletes are now taking supplements with L-arginine and L-citrulline to support the flow of blood and oxygen to the skeletal muscle. These supplements can be dangerous. These are used to facilitate the removal of exercise-induced lactic acid build-up, which reduces fatigue and recovery time.

Supplements can help restore this nitric oxide loop, allowing for better workouts and faster recovery from workouts. With nitric oxide deficiencies due to aging, inactivity, smoking, high cholesterol, fatty diets, and lack of healthy foods, increasing your nitric oxide levels can help increase your energy, vitality and overall wellness. The basic adage of eating well and staying active all makes sense now.

SRM®Self-Applied Moves (Patent-pending)

The SRM self-applied movements are a series of coordinated, untwisting dynamic motions and stretches that result in the release of nitric oxide from the brain. We teach them so that they are time-efficient and built around the individual's busy schedule.

We teach it so that it only takes about 15-minutes. I treat many different types of patients of all ages, shapes and sizes. I treat *athletes, busy professionals, kids, and aging adults,* and they all can easily implement the movements into their daily routine to enjoy a myriad of health benefits.

The following list of instructions are for a few of the eleven (11) SRM Self-Applied Protocols that you must learn in order to increase nitric oxide production naturally at home. However, due to the complexity, I have only included the ones that you would be able to apply immediately with little risk. I remind you that it is virtually impossible to learn the protocols affectively without prior instructions and demonstrations. Only for the purposes of this book am I sharing a few, but we usually do not teach or show the protocols until you have been thoroughly evaluated and treated with SRM Physician-Applied Protocols:

Move #1 Cervical Thoracic Lumbar (CTL)

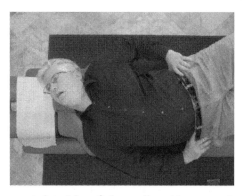

- You will start by lying on the foam roll vertically, with your entire spine on the roll—from tailbone to occiput (base of skull). Place both feet flat on the surface, with your knees bent.

- Place a hand on each hip and then place your head on the left or right side of the roll, taking caution not to rotate the head.

- Lengthen the right side of your spine by contracting the left musculature between the left pelvis and left rib cage. You should feel a shortening of your left side and a lengthening of the right side.

- Push back or flatten your back into the roll by performing a pelvic tilt. Take a breath in and then maximally exhale. When the air is fully exhaled, focus your attention on flattening the back further, while maintaining the left sided shortening and right sided lengthening.

- Repeat the stretch on the opposite side.

Move #3 Cranial Cervical Thoracic (CT)

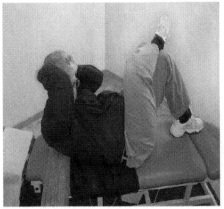
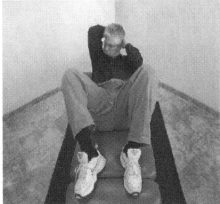

- Place the roll perpendicular to your spine, and lie on it at the mid-scapular level. Place both feet flat on the surface, with your knees bent. Take your right leg and cross it over the left knee.
- Take your left hand, reach behind the back of your head to find the midline point of the base of your skull, using the index finger. (This places the hand in the center of the occiput and slightly to the right of the midline.) Once this position is located, place your right hand over the left. Using both hands, now pull the head forward, so that the chin comes to the upper chest. Note: Avoid pulling the head too hard.
- Your left index finger remains fixed to its location at the back of the head. Now, drop your left elbow in towards the midline of the chest, pulling the head and chin with it.
- With your head now fully flexed, and your chin slightly turned to the right, the left arm gently pulls the head to the left. You should feel this stretch as a strong pull on the right side of the neck—from the occiput down to the thoracic spine—and along the right side into the trapezius muscle.
- Repeat the stretch on the opposite side.

Move #4 – Thoracic (T)

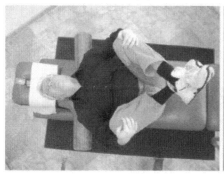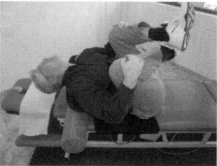

- Place the foam roll perpendicular to your spine, at the mid-scapular level. Place both feet flat on the surface, with knees bent.
- Grab your knees just below the kneecaps and pull both knees to your chest. Take a breath, and on the exhale, pull the knees strongly into the chest. (Maximal effectiveness is achieved with full exhalation of the breath.)
- Once your hips are at their maximal flexion (knees close as possible to the chest), the neck should be back into full extension.
- If you have minimal restriction flexing your hips, you should perform a pelvic tilt after the knees have been pulled into your chest.

Move #6 – Hip Pelvic (HP)

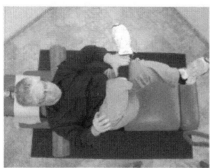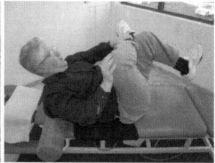

- Place the roll perpendicular to the spine, at the mid-scapular level. Place both feet flat on the surface, with knees bent.

- Take your right leg and place it on the left thigh about 3" below the kneecap.
- Now grab directly above your right ankle with your left hand.
- Place your right hand on your right knee. The leg should be perpendicular to the torso, and the right hand helps maintain this position.
- Take a breath, exhale, and pull both the right ankle and right knee toward the chest—as a fixed unit. The right knee should not drift laterally. The left thigh helps in this movement by pushing the right leg toward the chest. Note that the left foot will leave the surface as this occurs.
- Repeat the stretch on the opposite side.

Move #8 – Seated Hip Pelvic Lumbar (SHPL) (No foam roll required)

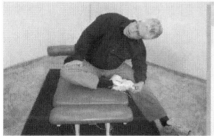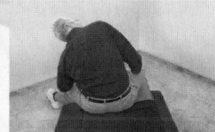

- Sit on a flat, raised surface with your hips perpendicular to that surface. The height of the surface varies depending on the leg length. Your outreached leg should reach the floor if possible.
- Take the right foot and place it on the surface with the knee flat and bent at ninety degrees or less. The left leg is off the surface, straight and outstretched to the left, the left heel upon the ground, toes up.
- Turn your upper body to the right.
- Place your right hand on your right thigh. The left hand is placed under your right foot. The two arms are used to direct your torso downward along your left side.
- Take a breath, exhale slowly, and lower your body to the left, following the line of the right leg. With each successive breath and

exhalation, you attempt to lower your torso downward along the left thigh. It may take several exhalations to achieve the greatest possible lowering for that day.

- Repeat the stretch on the opposite side.

Move #10– Thigh/Pelvis Junction (TPJ)

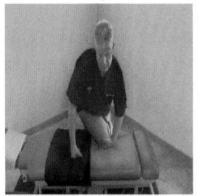 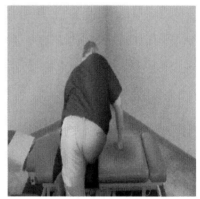

- You start by locating a surface in your home that is from 3-4 feet off the ground; firm is preferred over a soft surface.
- Face the surface square, and place your right thigh on the surface with the knee bent. The heel of the right foot should be placed to the outside of the opposite thigh.
- The left hand reaches for the right knee, pulling the knee further to the left side. It's important to observe that the right hip will try to follow the knee to the left. This is the motion that must be resisted. Where the thigh and pelvis meet is called the hip. The object of this move is to separate these structures.
- With the thigh pulled to the left, bend forward slightly from the waist. This should create more tension at that thigh/pelvic junction.
- Start turning the lower body to the right, with emphasis on starting the motion from the thigh/pelvic junction. This movement takes patience and practice in order to fully appreciate the tension in this area.
- Hold the position for 30 seconds or to tolerance.
- Repeat this movement on the opposite side

SRM for the Athlete

For the athlete, this means tighter muscles, poorer recovery, decrease performance, or increased effort to reach maximal performance. The SRM reverses this cycle of stress in as little time as 12 minutes. It's important to introduce the SRM into a daily regimen of treatment to keep tight muscles from moving onto a more difficult phase of treatment. The SRM provides a competitive advantage for professional level competition or general sport. We notice improvements in workouts, improved or greater endurance, and faster recovery times.

SRM for the Busy Professional

For the busy professional, the hardest thing to handle is the time to implement what we will teach you. That is why both groups of self-applied protocols take about 15 minutes each to complete. The SRM can relieve the buildup of mental, physical and chemical stresses that ultimately lead to physical pain and other health issues. Getting more oxygen to your brain and increasing the release of nitric oxide can have huge implications on your ability to think on your feet and to be mentally prepared for whatever life throws at you.

The body is connected to the mind through breathing. When we surrender the mind using the exhaled breath, the body can return to its perfect basic form and function. Holding an SRM allows a novice patient time to connect body and mind and to relax.

The SRM restores normal nitric oxide levels, and consequently, restores vascular tone. In addition, because the SRM moves produce an acute stress, we may be improving the chemistries that help produce both an inflammatory and a pro-immune response. The patients experience is a euphoric feeling, (which is actually the forgotten norm), and the return of all the positive aspects of good physiology. Second, by addressing the right side of contracture or twist, the SRM improves the margins, making it more difficult for forms of stress to have its effect on the body.

Four ways diet can naturally boost Nitric Oxide:

1) BEET IT… Eat more Beets – Juice beets if you don't like raw or cooked beets, but use organic beets and include the roots, and even the leaves. Beets naturally boost the production of nitric oxide in the body and support energy levels. Beets contain large amounts of nitrates found within the vegetable. Beetroot juice also supports immunity and helps to protect against certain cancers.

2) Consume Hawthorn Extract – Hawthorn is used to prevent heart disease because it prevents plaque from coating the arterial walls, acts as a calcium-channel blocker which protects the endothelial cells that line our blood vessels, and secretes nitric oxide.

3) Exercise Every Day – When you are physically active, the heart has to pump harder to supply more oxygen to the body, and the additional pressure against the arterial walls, from more blood passing through, causes more nitric oxide to be released.

4) East Fruits and Nuts - They are two of the best sources of these amino acids, but amino acids also exist in meat and dairy. However, the antioxidants in fruits and nuts also protect the nitric oxide that is created by eating these foods.

While sports companies would have you believe you have to take a supplement supposed to build muscle, and your doctor may recommend a pharmaceutical drug to prevent heart disease, the best way to boost your body's own production of nitric oxide, and enjoy some better sex while you are at it, is to make sure your body is not in the twist and implement the physician-applied and self-applied protocols.

Self-Applied…..Personal Hyperbaric Chamber

As with the Stress Relief Method and Lois Laynee Breathing Method, there are doctor-applied protocols and self-applied protocols. In cases of advanced trauma and/or for serious wound healing (and a few other cases where there is medical necessity), we recommend home hyperbaric therapy treatments. We provide our patients with a variety to choose from to make sure our patients purchase or lease the proper one suited for their individual needs. We offer suggestions on how to have your health insurance carrier cover the home chamber and financing may be available.

Home portable chamber, come in various different makes, models and sizes. They are usually referred to as "personal hyperbaric chambers." This is in reference to the lower pressure that these chambers operate at as compared to the hard steel commercial grade chambers.

In the USA, these "personal hyperbaric chambers" are categorized by the FDA as CLASS II medical devices and requires a prescription in order to purchase one or take treatments. Personal hyperbaric chambers are only FDA approved to reach 1.3 ATA. While hyperbaric chamber distributors and manufacturers cannot supply a chamber in the USA with any form of elevated oxygen delivery system, a physician can write a prescription to combine the two modalities, as long as there is a prescription for both hyperbaric and oxygen.

The most common option, but it is not approved by FDA at this time, is to utilize an oxygen concentrator, which typically delivers 85–90% oxygen. Because of the high circulation of air through the chamber, the total concentration of oxygen in the chamber never exceeds 25% as there is a risk of fire. Oxygen is never fed directly into the soft chambers but is rather introduced via a gas line and mask directly to the patient.

The FDA-approved, oxygen concentrators for human consumption are regularly monitored for purity (+/- 1%) and flow (10 to 15 liters per minute outflow pressure). The units have an audible alarm that will sound if the purity drops below 80%. The soft chambers are approved by the FDA for the treatment of altitude sickness, but are commonly used for other "off-label" purposes. Soft chambers are safe when used as directed.

Chapter 8

Motivation and Determination

Two of the most important things that you need to keep the Self-Sustainable Healthy Lifestyle Program alive – even more important than an instructor or a doctor – are your own motivation and determination. You have to be motivated to do well, and you have to be determined to take stock in the situation. If you are overweight and looking to shed pounds, no gym instructor anywhere in the world can help you if you don't take adequate measures to secure consistency.

Even if you are sick and are looking at treatment, no doctor can help if you aren't committed to following the treatment program to the end, whether it's taking the medication at the right time, abstaining from toxic foods, or doing the recommended exercises.

Even God doesn't help those who don't help themselves.

So, before even thinking of going ahead with a fitness or a healthy lifestyle program, the one thing you need to be sure of is your own commitment to it.

You have to make sure you will be motivated to carry on the program until the very end. The best way to do it, of course, is to focus and concentrate on the end result. If you are planning to enter into a weight loss program, you could think about the great body, better sex, and more energy you will have if you follow the program. Or, if you have some cardiac ailment right now, think about how sticking to the right medical program, specific for you, will make you feel after a few months. You will be able to do things as before, or maybe even better, and your life will be so much richer.

The best way to keep yourself motivated is to always think about what is to come. Think about the results of your efforts. The efforts you need to put in won't seem so very difficult then.

Choosing the Proper Program

It is highly important to choose the proper program right from the start. Do not guess! Or YOU WILL FAIL!

The health and fitness industry is probably the most saturated industry in the world today. Part of the reason for that is people try out one program and they fail because of their own lack of determination. Then they think the program is worthless and try another. What the health and fitness industry don't tell people is that they are failing mostly because they are not able to resolve themselves to stick to one program. They will also probably fail with this one because their minds are like rolling stones - it doesn't matter, because presently they are spending thousands of dollars on buying many other unneeded products.

Unfortunately, that's the way it works because the health and fitness industry is saturated. So what do you do when you are looking at a program for yourself? If it is a health treatment program, your choice is simple. You just go to a doctor that you have faith in – usually your family physician – and then do as they say. But the issue is very much complicated if you are looking for a viable fitness program. What do you use to stay fit – diet, exercise, aerobics, calisthenics? This should be part of the real healthcare system, where your physician would discuss and interest you in these variables for improving your life.

Researching on the Internet is not the answer. What you will find mostly is articles full of sales pitch, written by people who are trying to promote their own product. They won't have any qualms in painting some other perfectly good product with a negative color if they can improve the impression of their own product. The world gobbles it up, so it works.

You can also join a health and fitness club. We offer many different classes to our patients in our gym facility. This is a great place to meet people who are conscious about their fitness, and they won't mind giving you great advice. Many fitness clubs have their own libraries, too, so you could find a lot of educational material in them.

When you get the books on what you are thinking about, take time out and read them. Read them mainly to understand what you will have to do, how much time you will have to devote, what equipment you will need, whether you will be able to do what is mentioned, what the results will be, and how soon you will get them, etc. These facts will help you decide whether you want to be with the program.

Don't trust anybody when it comes to deciding a fitness program for you. Most people will have commercial interests. Some well-meaning souls will give you advice, too, but they may be limited in their knowledge, and a professional medical team should be considered instead. It is best to speak with impartial experts, like your doctor, or read books and form an initial decision. Of course, you need to speak with a qualified person before making your eventual decision about what program to take.

Chapter 9

Take Control of Your Fitness

Exercising doesn't have to be a leg burning, lung collapsing, high-cardio session or a sweat-filled weight lifting experience where you feel pain or hurt. Approaching your health from a functional point of view just has to include activity, and the more variety you have, the more likely you'll actually look forward to physical activity.

So let's first lay the foundation for an active life. Let's go over the benefits of exercise, and how it can improve all areas of your life.

The most obvious benefit of being active is it's a surefire way to maintain a healthy weight or reduce weight. Moving burns calories. Even the most casual type of movement burns calories, so you're sure to get that benefit no matter what your mobility or physical condition.

Regular physical activity will help you mange, or greatly reduce, the risk of contracting various health conditions and diseases. A few examples of these diseases and disorders include: osteoporosis, arthritis, depression, heart disease, type 2 diabetes, stroke and certain types of cancer.

Exercising is a form of treatment for depression, and it also helps you feel more relaxed and happier. Various brain chemicals are released by exercise that lifts your spirit and gives you a more positive outlook. Once you get over the fact that you don't always feel like you have the energy to be active, you can embrace the reality that after exercising (especially when providing your body with the appropriate fuel), you will feel more energetic. In addition, when you increase your heart rate on a daily basis, you'll have a long-term flow of energy.

If you are having trouble getting to sleep or actually sleeping...

EXERCISE! Getting active regularly encourages a quicker and deeper sleep, when completed at least 4-5 hours before bedtime. We will discuss the benefits to getting a proper night's sleep in a later chapter.

On the relationship side, regular physical activity promotes a happier sex life. Various aspects come into play for this benefit: the energy boost will get you feeling in the mood, and all those feel good hormones released during exercise (endorphins, dopamine, adrenaline, and serotonin) will work synergistically to make you feel happy and confident. This relates to an increased libido. Of course, there's the toned and buffed body, along with a greater range of motion, that you'll enjoy all throughout the day.

Physical Activity That Suits You

Exercising in the great outdoors has the added benefit of soaking in the natural surroundings. Besides joining in directed fitness classes and going to the gym, there are many ways to get more exercise into your day, including exercising in the great outdoors.

Integrating just a few of these exercises will not only help you reap the benefits of exercise, but will also create a lifestyle full of fun, new experiences, and with a deeper inner awareness.

Here are a few ways to incorporate cardiovascular activities, with little or no equipment, which you can start today:

- **Ride a Bike** –Riding your bike instead of driving is a popular way to get some exercise while going about your daily activities. And it's great for the environment, too!
- **Climb Stairs** – Add some physical activity to your day by choosing to take a flight of stairs instead of an escalator or elevator. Running upstairs is an amazing exercise; but downhill

running or decline stairs is bad for the knees, and you will need to be careful if you start to feel knee pain.

- **Dancing** - Go out dancing! Almost every culture in the world has its own form of dancing. It is fun and dancing is an incredible workout that can burn a lot of calories.
- **Skip** – It's not just for kids anymore. Skipping provides an excellent cardio workout that provides a number of benefits, including improved coordination, enhanced bone density, high calorie burning, and core muscle strengthening.
- **Ski** – Not only is skiing great for your health and body tone, it also helps brighten the winter's negative side effects.
- **Walk or Run** – A quick walk can be just as beneficial as running, without the wear and tear on your body if you are a beginner. For an added benefit, park further away from the store. Those extra steps add up to great health!
- **Jump on a Trampoline** – A small exercise trampoline provides an easy source of high-cardio activity without the high-impact and can be used 5-10 minutes a day. And it's a lot of fun!
- **Stretching** - While stretching your body, you extend and lengthen your joints, increasing flexibility and resulting in better control of your movements throughout the day.
- **Weight Lifting** – Gives a greater ability to build stronger muscles.
- **Pilates/Yoga** –Although there are some differences between Pilates and Yoga, they both focus on increasing muscle tone and flexibility.
- **Bodyweight Training** – Through lunges, squats, crunches and push-ups, this uses the weight and movement of your own body to tone and build strong muscles.

Say Hello to Mother Nature and Go Camping

If you regularly go camping, you'll enjoy dozens of significant health benefits. Here are some obvious ones:

Fresh Air - When you spend time near a lot of trees, you take in more oxygen. That feeling of happiness that you get, when you take your first breath of air at the campground, isn't all in your head—well, technically it is, but it's a release of serotonin from the extra oxygen. Your body can function with less strain when there's plenty of oxygen. That's not the only benefit of fresh air. Research shows that some time outdoors can improve your blood pressure, improve digestion, and give your immune system an extra boost. When you spend a few days outside, you get some serious health benefits from the extra oxygen and low levels of pollutants.

Socialization - Camping alone is plenty of fun, but if you bring along a friend or family member, you'll enjoy a unique experience together that will help you keep a healthy, happy relationship. According to research published in the American Journal of Public Health, socializing can extend your lifespan and delay memory problems. Apart from the medical benefits, a few close relationships make life more fun. Invite a few friends on your next trip out.

Improved Mood - Regular campers will often talk about how the first few days back from a trip seem happier. This isn't without merit; spending some time outside in the sunlight can even out the levels of melatonin in your brain. Melatonin is the chemical that makes you feel tired and can induce feelings of depression, so by camping, you can enjoy better overall moods during and after your trip.

Less Stress - Camping also allows you to cope with stress. Stress can negatively affect your health in just about every way possible, and you're putting much less strain on your mental and physical faculties by giving yourself some stress-free time at the campsite. The lack of stress is related to the rise in oxygen levels, higher levels of serotonin, and managed levels of melatonin mentioned above. There's also an emotional component at work here, since it's harder to be annoyed or angry when you're doing something that you enjoy.

Exercise - Let's not forget the most obvious benefit of camping: you're spending a lot of time performing physical activities. Even if you're taking a fishing trip, you're burning more calories than you'd burn sitting around an office, and if you hike or bike, you're performing cardiovascular exercise that will help keep your heart and lungs healthy. Your activity levels will vary, but hiker's burn anywhere from 120-300 calories per hour, bikers burn 300-500 calories per hour, and fly fishing can burn up to 200 calories per hour. No wonder you work up such an appetite during a long camping trip.

Sunshine - Sunshine feels great on your skin, and there's an evolutionary reason for that. When you're out in direct sunlight, you're taking on a lot of Vitamin D, which allows your body to absorb calcium and phosphorous.

A Good Night's Sleep - Assuming that you've got decent camping gear, you'll fall fast asleep after a day full of outdoor activities. Sleep has an effect on all of your body processes and can reduce inflammation, improve your cardiovascular system, and help you stay alert. Many campers report better sleep cycles when they return from a trip.

Good Food - If you pack s'mores, you're not seeing any particularly solid health benefits in this department. However, if you're fond of fishing and hunting, you'll likely eat a large amount of protein and healthy fats on your camping trip. You won't get any preservatives or unnatural ingredients in a fresh lake-caught fish, and all of the exercise on your trip will help your digestion and allow you to rest.

New Challenges – Trust me. No two camping trips are exactly the same, and that's a great thing. Studies from the University of Texas and University of Michigan show that new experiences keeps the brain healthy. New activities that are both physically and intellectually stimulating have the greatest effect on brain health, and camping fits both of these criteria perfectly.

Meditation - When you go camping, don't forget to turn off your cell phone, the tablet, and the laptop computer. Shut the chaos off. Close your eyes, sit back and just breathe. Try to disconnect and enjoy the simplicity of the natural experiences and peace that camping provides. This is a perfect time to practice your Layne Restorative Breathing Method and the SRM Self-Applied Protocols. This is a general tip to help you enjoy the experience: if you're willing to enjoy your surroundings without any outside distractions, it will increase your lifespan. The Mayo Clinic reports that meditation may improve a number of serious medical conditions by simply increasing self-awareness and giving a person a stress-reduction tool. If you suffer from depression, fatigue, heart disease, or even allergies, research shows that camping can improve your overall health.

In an ideal world, your body should get at least 30 minutes of energizing cardiovascular activity every day, along with a 30-40 minute strength training session and a lengthening flexibility or patterning (SRM and LOIS Breathing) routine of another 20 minutes. If you commit to this you'll see and feel the great results of your commitment on the inside and out. However, this can also be a goal to achieve as you make your progress towards a health-focused lifestyle.

Take A Slow Start

The key is to start slow. When you start your health and fitness program at a slow pace, you are much more comfortable with it, and you get used to it. You should not feel totally destroyed after the workout in the beginning. Obviously, once you get stronger, you will be able to push to higher levels of fitness.

When you are embarking on your new fitness regimen, don't make that huge mistake of taking long strides right from the start. This is especially important when you are going to do things your own way. For example, if you are going to go jogging each morning, don't plan on jogging for an hour right from the first day.

Start slow – maybe just walk instead for 20 to 35 minutes the first day. You probably haven't exercised in a long time; therefore, you might also have a problem with stamina. When your stamina increases, you will be able to exert yourself for longer. But if you think of going full force right from the start, you will be exhausted to the point of giving up.

I also suggest staying away from downhill walking, jogging or running when first starting out. The downhill run will play havoc on the knees because your knees won't be ready for the deceleration stresses associated with downhill activity. Instead try inclines and bleachers or staircases.

The same applies when you are trying to go on a diet. You could not possibly give up all your favorite foods all at once. This will actually put you into depression and make you quickly give up. Foods are chemicals, and our body becomes accustomed to the chemicals it comes in contact with. Simply removing the chemicals will often cause depression. Depression releases a hormone known as cortisol. Cortisol – also known as the stress hormone – will make you mentally weak and vulnerable. Depression also taxes the adrenal glands, and I estimate that 80% of Americans are either in Adrenal Fatigue or even Adrenal Failure.

Instead, you could start by giving up a few of the unhealthy foods; work them out of your schedule slowly. Even when you are on a strict diet, it is advisable to have at least one favorite "cheat" meal per week, so that you don't feel too stressed out. In fact, you will be looking forward to that special meal each week.

Chapter 10

<u>YOU</u> Have to Take Control of Your Fitness

Targeting the Right Parts of the Body

One of the biggest problems in following health and fitness programs arise when people don't know what they should be doing. Most of the time people do not know exactly what their body needs, and often it is the exercises that they are doing that make the problems worse.

There are hundreds of different machines and pieces of equipment that are confusing and often complicated to use. This is why we use the FMS, so there is never any guessing. We know, and you will know, exactly what functional exercise pattern you should be doing.

The FMS is the starting point for every exercise program we use, and we re-screen our patients to make sure they are improving. The FMS keeps our patients from doing things that they shouldn't be doing. Not just that, patients often exert themselves in doing worthless exercises that are ineffective and can cause more problems.

In fact, some people try prioritizing their fitness regimens. They use the FMS to determine what to do first, and then focus their energies on that. When their FMS has improved, they move on to another set of exercise progressions. Such focused attention works very well, especially in today's world when we are cramped for time and don't want to waste effort.

If you are joining a gym after a long time of physical inactivity, you will find that you will need to focus on building your stamina first. For that, you might be asked to work on the treadmill or an exercise bike initially. Once you have built up your system's capabilities, they will ask you to slowly start with resistance training. You might be focusing on one particular aspect for a few weeks, then move on to another area. This actually helps you – you are working out in a way that your body needs.

If you were to go all out at once, you would end up stressing your body to the max, and this could be disastrous to your long-term planning. You might stretch your body so extensively that you will not be able to lift a finger. When that happens, people don't stick to their fitness plans.

The mistake isn't the program itself – it's probably the way in which you approach it.

The Deadlift (King of the Build)

My favorite types of exercise programs are functional workouts, and my favorite exercise is the basic and good, old-fashioned Deadlift.

When performed correctly, the deadlift is one of the best exercises to build total body mass. The deadlift strengthens all the major muscle groups and develops tone in the core.

In my experience as an athlete and physician, and based on the years of results that I have personally witnessed, the deadlift, when performed correctly, builds unparalleled mass and strengthens all the major muscle groups in the body.

Yes, I know that many squat fanatics will argue that the squat is the best exercise for building mass, and they are not wrong. Yes, the squat will increase strength and size better than any other exercise. We include squats in almost everyone's weight training program that we prescribe. However, pound for pound and taking safety into account, the deadlift, in my opinion, builds the body more effectively than any other exercise and it's a totally functional exercise.

The deadlift is done by simply grasping a weight, usually a free-weight bar, and lifting up until you're standing up with the bar hanging in front of you, arms extended. We use kettle bells, heavy bands, sand bags, and other types of resistance apparatuses to work the deadlift. This may sound simple, enough but the deadlift must be taught to do properly for the best outcomes, and most people do not know how to do it properly.

The Benefits of Deadlifts

1. Fat Burning - Alwyn Cosgrove, a fitness author and extremely notable professional fitness trainer, recently wrote about a study where:

"Overweight subjects were assigned to three groups:

1. Diet-only
2. Diet plus aerobics
3. Diet plus aerobics plus weights

Group 1, or the *diet only* group, lost 14.6 pounds in 12 weeks. Group 2, or the *diet and aerobic* group, lost 15.6 pounds in 12 weeks (training was three times a week starting at 30 minutes and progressing to 50 minutes over the 12 weeks). Group 3, or the *weight training* group, lost the most at 21.1 pounds (44% and 35% more than diet and diet/aerobic groups respectively)."

The end result of this study was that just the addition of aerobic training did not result in significant fat loss any more than just dieting alone. Only a few pound differentiated between Groups 1 and 2, as opposed to Group 3 that incorporated lifting weights and resistance training. Group 3 burned more fat than just dieting or dieting with cardio exercise alone.

2. Improves Posture - The first step in the proper deadlift is to tighten or create tone in the core. Deadlifting increases your core strength and adds to core stability. Deadlifting targets all of the muscles responsible for your proper posture control and strengthens your back muscles, which keep your back straighter during regular daily activities.

3. More Muscles Utilized - Recent research has proved that the deadlift utilizes more muscles in the body at one time than any other exercise, including the squat. The deadlift engages all of the major muscle groups and tones the core. If you should do one exercise, this is the one to do. The deadlift works your whole body, the upper and lower, including all the major back muscles, and most notably, the core.

4. Functional for Real Life – Take other lifting exercises, like the straight bar bench press, for example, the likelihood you're going to do anything like that in real life is slim. Although the bench press is important, it doesn't have the direct impact on your daily functioning like the deadlift. The deadlift develops the muscles you need to actually carry something, like a heavy bucket of water, or bags of groceries, or to lift a wheel barrel.

5. Safe - The deadlift, when performed properly, is one of the safest weightlifting exercises that can be done. Unlike the bench press or the squat, you aren't going to get pinned under the weight or have to worry about falling over backwards. If you get into trouble in the deadlift, you simply just drop the weight. And although you should have a partner while working out, you do not have to have a spotter to perform a deadlift exercise.

6. Grip Strength - One of the biggest benefits from doing deadlifts is the ability to build grip strength. Your fingers and hands are literally the only things connecting you to the weight. Your forearms work incredibly hard as you lift the weight. Your finger grip actually keeps the weight from falling out of your hands. Subsequently, your grip strength increases.

7. Increases Testosterone and Growth Hormone – If you do at least three sets of deadlifts with a significant weight (half to three fourths your body weight), you can increase the amount of testosterone and growth hormone produced by your body. Your body uses testosterone to increase muscle growth and improve tissue repair. Growth Hormone, which is produced by your pituitary gland in your brain, promotes tissue healing, bone strength and muscle growth, as well as fat loss.

8. Low cost for effectiveness - A lot of exercises can require plenty of equipment, locations, special shoes or clothing. The deadlift does not require much of anything. It just requires a weight - a bar, heavy kettlebells, or dumbbells.

9. Cardiovascular improvement - The deadlift improves cardio vascularity by requiring the whole body to hold the tone during the lift, which requires the heart to pump more blood.

10. Injury Prevention – The deadlift can help prevent injuries by increasing the strength of the soft tissues that surround the spine, as well as strengthening the critical tendons and ligaments that protect the joints. Supporting the joints with strong ligaments, tendons, and muscles is crucial to preventing injury and correcting asymmetries in flexion and extension movements.

Involve Your Friends

Your friends could be quite instrumental in making you stick with your fitness plan. Many health and fitness advocators say that if you work out with a friend, you do much better. If you have someone to go to the gym with you, or diet with you, or accompany you on your morning jogs, you stick much better to your routine and to the program itself. They could be the support system you need and could greatly motivate you. Friends make working out much more fun.

There are many reasons why it works. The main reason is that boredom does not creep in, especially when you have a friend to work out with. We aren't bored when we are with our friends, right? Also, there might actually be a healthy competition sparked between the two of you. You might want to see who can lift better weights, who can jog more, who can diet better, etc. All this keeps you highly involved in your fitness program and positively motivated.

In fact, if you have a friend to accompany you in your health and fitness programs, you will actually start looking forward to that time of the day when you can work out with them. It is FUN!

Chapter 11

Motivation and Progress Are A MUST

One very important thing for you to do, when you are on a fitness program, is to keep track of your progress, which will keep you motivated. Doing this on a daily, weekly and monthly basis will keep you highly motivated, especially when you are able to see the dramatic changes that you have envisioned for yourself.

The Five Main Points to Live By:

1. Punctual - shows respect and consideration
1. Present - You're mentally present for communication
2. Caring - You are concerned about people or task
3. Compassionate - You do not want to hurt anyone
4. Accountable - You hold yourself to what you say and do

So, when you are on a diet program, weigh yourself often. When you are jogging, check how many steps you can climb without breathing heavily. When you are working out at the gym, keep checking your abs and chest. When you are on a program to improve your blood sugar level or your blood pressure, keep monitoring yourself. In fact, go for more frequent physical checkups just to see how well you are progressing.

Humans are very much result-oriented creatures. We want to see facts and figures – we want to see things as raw as they can be. This is the reason why charting your progress consistently can help immensely.

When you see your waist size coming down from 38" to 36", when you see that you can get into skimpier shorts or skinny jeans, and when you see that you are closer to touching your toes than before, you become proud and pleased with yourself. You see that your efforts are paying off. This keeps the fire burning.

Initially, you will want to monitor yourself quite often. Your family may even mock you for that. But it doesn't matter. You need to know where you are heading. So keep looking as much as you want. It is only when you are in love with your body that you will think of doing something for it. No one loves your body more than you, so the responsibility of making it fitter and healthier is entirely on you.

Don't Be Lazy...Don't make an excuse...Get in the Gym

One of the ways in which you can motivate yourself to keep working out is by simply taking the effort to go to the gym. Research shows that most people who quit their gyms don't do it because the exercises are too stressful; they do it just because they don't want to make the trip to the gym! If you have joined a gym before, you know this feeling. You don't mind the exercises, but you struggle with getting up early, putting on your gym clothes and heading out to the gym.

Try this: If you don't want to go to the gym on one particular day, tell yourself that you will just warm up a bit on the treadmill and then leave. Tell yourself that you won't do anything that needs too much exertion. When you convince yourself that way, you are likelier to head to the gym. And then, when you get there, get your butt moving. Getting there is the first battle.

But when you are there, you will see a change happening in your way of thinking. When you see all those people diligently working out, you will get motivated, too. And when you start out on the treadmill, you will find that your stamina is building. When that happens, you will tell yourself that you could try one more exercise. You might go on to the exercise bike. That may induce you to go to the weights and then the resistance training and so on. Sooner than you think, you will find that you have had your complete workout!

Studies show that this approach works in 90% of the cases: i.e. 90% of the people who come to the gym reluctantly, thinking that they will only work out for 5 minutes, end up working out their full routine.

The same idea applies with other things. If you are feeling lazy about going jogging, convince yourself by saying that it is only for a few minutes. You might tell yourself that you would do nothing more than one lap around the park. But when you are into it, you feel that you might as well complete the whole thing.

Sticking to Your Health and Fitness Program

Given the large rate of failure of health and fitness programs worldwide, it is easy to see why anyone will have apprehension when they try to get into such a program all by themselves. They are bound to think whether or not such programs will work for them. Even when you join a gym, however enthusiastic you are, somewhere in the corner of your mind, you wonder how long you will be attending the gym. These damaging feelings start when you haven't even had your first workout or stepped into the gym!

This happens universally. People join health and fitness programs only to leave them after a few days, weeks or months. It is their own weakness that makes them quit, but the world doesn't waste any time in jumping to the conclusion that something is not quite right with the program.

One of the best things you can do for yourself is to condition your mind into thinking positively about the program you are about to join. Don't keep any space for pessimism. There is no reason why you should think that the program won't work for you. Think that it will work. Think about all the benefits you will get because of that. Think about your sexier body shape, your healthier heart, your improved physical capacity, and you will want to carry through.

Think about how you will become a better individual. Think about how you will be able to travel to all those places when you are healthier. Think about how your bank balance will improve because you will become more productive. Think about how you will get better prospects at work because you are healthier. An improving professional life is what sets most of us thinking.

Also think about how you will be able to spend more quality time with your friends and family. Think how you won't be the one sitting in the corner when they are having fun right in front of you. You will be able to join in the merriment as well. If nothing works, take a look at your children and grandchildren. Wouldn't you like to be with them for a longer time? Wouldn't you like to see how they progress in life under your guidance?

Reward Yourself

Time and again, reward yourself for your achievements. However, don't reward yourself with a food treat; that will only make matters worse. In any case, we are too much fixated on food. When we are happy, the first thing that comes to our mind is a treat that involves the worst kinds of unhealthy foods possible. And this is what brings on most of the health problems that we face today. We could do much better from a health point of view if we cured our fixation with food.

But you could always give yourself a healthy incentive. You could go on a trip, for example. You could take a break from work and simply hang out at home, watching DVDs. Or you could cook a healthy meal all by yourself at home if that interests you.

One way to reward yourself for a great achievement is to take a vacation or break from the habits that brought you down in the first place. Change is good. When you start to feel better, you may try something new. Often, when we go on vacations, we walk more or we are more active because we are not in our normal mundane patterns.

However, the best incentive is looking in the mirror. When you see the improved shape you are in, you will want to congratulate yourself. In fact, you should keep some of your old photos for comparison. When you know how well you have turned out so far, you will want to go all the way. You will feel that it is quite possible for you to take further steps.

Go shopping - Buy clothes that fit your newly reworked body. You will be so happy about buying jeans that are two sizes smaller. You will feel you have achieved something special.

You have to understand something here. When you measure yourself at home and see that you have reduced, you are happy; you become much happier when you reward yourself for it. When you buy smaller jeans, you see the practical connotations of your fitness program. You actually see the benefits. This is what motivates you to keep working on you in the future. If you see these benefits and then begin rewarding yourself for it, you will see that you are able to push yourself toward better health and fitness achievements.

Go Hunting and Fishing - You always knew hunting and fishing were good for your health, but now science can back it up. Angling can improve the condition of your heart, body and mind.

Some of the health benefits of fishing include: improving muscle dexterity and strength through reeling, casting, and walking; absorbing fresh air and Vitamin D while you're outside; and relaxing your mind by unplugging from the high-stress path you're on. Walking around the forest, or the rugged terrain, will provide an incredible work out. If you are lucky enough to bag an animal or catch a whopper, you will certainly have a workout cleaning and hauling your prize.

Anyone who hunts or fishes experiences some form of unexplainable satisfaction from being in the outdoors. Many hunters and fishermen report feeling closer to nature when they are outdoors. Studies have even shown that hunting and fishing increases a man's so-called "love hormone." It may have to do with the negative ions outside, the fresh air, the feeling of freedom, and most likely, the lack of technology.

Take regular weekend trips or breaks to the great outdoors. Waiting for that big trip is actually counterproductive; smaller get-a-ways are way healthier and break up the monotony better. The average person is sitting still for approximately 9.3 hours per day. The average American family puts in more than 11 hours of work per week - more now than they did in 1979. And get this - 20% of Americans work more than 50 hours per week and take 7 vacation days a year.

Benefits to your heart - Walking to your favorite fishing hole can increase heart rate for improved cardiovascular. Deep sea and other types of fishing can be strenuous when fighting and reeling in a big fish.

Benefits to your brain - Simply just unplugging from daily stresses can recharge your brain, giving you better focus or clarity. One Japanese study measured the difference between people who spend a few hours a day in a wooded area versus those who spent the same amount of time in the city. The nature group had lower blood pressure, pulse, and cortisol.

Benefits to your body – The body is adaptable and the constant crossing of the midline, while doing outdoor activities, helps with coordination and balance. Fresh, clean air, (air with lower amounts of air pollution) makes being outside great for our lungs. Finally, we can't forget Vitamin D, which is a very important vitamin. It is increased by exposure to the sun and protects the body from heart disease, muscle development, and brain function.

They say that the average American child is in front of some type of screen or monitor 7 hours a day. Being outdoors has been proven to improve distance vision and decrease nearsightedness. There is ample research that has shown that being outside greatly reduces ADHD in children.

The physical benefits of hunting and fishing are obvious, but there are other benefits to getting in shape and maintaining a sound mind and body.

The Most Important Commodity That We Have Is TIME

You hear people say things like "time is a cruel mistress" or "time Flies!" and they are right. You only get about 30,000 days on earth, if you're lucky, and even Steve Jobs (CEO of Apple) could not buy more. So spend your time wisely. If you won't do it for yourself, then do it for someone else and donate your time.

The only thing more satisfying than good health is encouraging others to become healthier. I recommend giving back more than you receive. For me, I was driven to my non-profit - Keep It Simple-Make It Fun (KISMIF).

KISMIF is a recreational therapy program that provides the opportunity for disabled, and non-disabled, individuals to socialize together in a friendly, leisurely setting. Family members and friends alike have the chance to paddle a canoe, hike a mountain, relax on the beach, or just sit and talk around a fire.

As the name implies, the Keep It-Simple Make It Fun program was established due to the low number of programs for disabled individuals and the lack of funding for the programs that do exist. The whole basis of KISMIF is to get back to the basics in life by enjoying the great outdoors in a friendly, warm, and relaxed setting.

The satisfaction a person gets from sharing Mother Nature is a wonderful feeling. Sharing food you may have hunted with others, who either want or need low-fat, high-protein game meat, is a great feeling. "Many a man has found himself while in the service of others." I don't know who said that, but it works for me. I take great pride and satisfaction sharing all that I have with my family and friends, especially my friends in KISMIF.

It is not generosity that drives me to share; it is selfishness. I love the feeling I get from sharing and helping others, so it makes me feel good and I am not ashamed to admit it. It also provides a good example for those around me and encourages them to share and help. Sometimes, a positive action can inspire other positive actions, and so on and so on. Why not do your part and make people and places around you better than when you found them.

Final Healthy Thoughts

The best way to make any health and fitness program work is to simply make it Fun. Having fun, and enjoying the process, makes it so much more enjoyable and rewarding in the end. If you have the right motivation and determination, you will keep yourself pepped up so that you follow through till the end. You will feel better and see yourself in a newer light. That will really help this highly important task you are embarking upon.

Chapter 12

The importance of A Good Night's Sleep

You may be wondering why I would include this sleep chapter in a Self-Sustaining Healthy Lifestyle. Well, the answer is easy; this whole book is about being self-sustainable. This means getting back to the basic essentials in life and doing the simple things to improve the quality of your life. I can't think of a more important subject to have in this book than proper sleep. There are literally hundreds, if not thousands, of articles or research papers that have established the many problems associated with not getting enough proper rest.

The lack of "good" sleep plays total havoc on your body. The lack of proper rest causes early aging, obesity, heart disease, poor body functioning, and depression. Even cancer has been linked to poor rest. So, I felt compelled to put information in this book about sleep - the effects of lack of sleep, and what I recommend to insure that you are getting the right amount of proper rest.

Sleep...Dream

Years ago, sleep was just something that we did to help rejuvenate our bodies. Over the years, through many studies, we have found that sleep is neither dormant nor passive. Our bodies are very much active, and depending on how we actually sleep determines our functioning process on a day-to-day basis. We are just beginning to understand the many ways that sleep is responsible for not only our physical health, but for our mental health as well.

Neurotransmitters, or nerve-signaling chemicals, are in charge when we are awake or asleep. They work on various types of nerve cells in our brains, producing additional chemicals that allow our brains to rest when we sleep, or keep our brain functional when awake.

There are many benefits to having a good night's sleep, including improved memory, feeling refreshed and focused, improved heart health, enhanced concentration, glowing skin, reduced inflammation, nurtured creativity, improved performance and stamina, sharpened attention, lower stress, and living longer.

When we sleep there are five different stages that we go through:

- Stage 1 – Falling Asleep
- Stage 2 – Brain Slow-down
- Stages 3 and 4 – Deep Sleep
- Stage 5 – Rapid Eye Movement (REM)

In each stage, both the body and the brain act differently. These stages cycle and repeat approximately every 90 minutes. While asleep, we spend 25 percent of our time in stages one, three and four, 25 percent in REM sleep, and 50 percent in stage two. In each stage, your brain and body will act differently; in some stages you will be immobilized, almost paralyzed, while other stages you are constantly moving.

We require all five stages for a healthy and balanced life, so developing proper sleep habits will ensure that you get each stage of sleep needed. So what are some of the characteristics of proper sleep, and why are they so important? Let's take a look:

- A regular sleep cycle supports your circadian (24-hour) rhythm.
- Sleep is responsible for a healthy immune system.
- The body does most of its growth, recovery and repair during sleep.
- During sleep, the metabolic rate and digestive system slows down.
- You might feel colder at night because the body temperature falls.

- Hormones produced during sleep regulate your appetite.
- Sleep is when the fertility, sex, and growth hormones are released.

Good sleep habits are vital if you want to be at your greatest and enjoy your life to the maximum.

How Much Sleep Do We Actually Need?

In each stage of our lives, we require different amounts of sleep. Infants usually require about 16 hours a day, teenagers need about 9 hours, and adults 7 to 8 hours a night. The amount of sleep a person requires will also increase, depending on the previous night. Sleep deprivation will eventually get caught up, but at what price? Reaction times, productivity, everyday decisions, decrease in memory, motor skills, and other functions may be impaired.

As people get older, although they still need as much sleep as they did as an early adult, they tend to sleep more lightly and for shorter time spans. About half of all people over 65 have frequent sleeping problems, which could include sleep apnea or insomnia, and deep sleep stages can either become very short or stop completely. This change may just be a normal part of aging, (I remember my grandmother saying she didn't need as much sleep as she used to) or it might result from medications associated with common medical problems that the elderly face.

The prevalent habit of "burning the candle at both ends" has led to an increase in sleep deprivation, so much so, that what was considered "abnormal sleepiness" is now pretty much the norm. Sleep deprivation is dangerous. Let's take a look at, for example, truck drivers. How many accidents are caused because truck drivers have a rigid schedule to keep, and from time to time, the proper amount of sleep just doesn't fit into their schedule? Many more than should be allowed. The National Sleep Foundation says: "If you have trouble keeping your eyes focused, if you can't stop yawning, or if you can't remember driving the last few miles, you are probably too drowsy to drive safely."

In order for our nervous systems to work properly, sleep is a necessity. Not enough sleep causes drowsiness, hinders our concentration, reduces the ability to properly solve math equations, diminishes physical performance, and leads to impaired memory. The continuation of sleep deprivation may lead to more drastic symptoms, such as mood swings or hallucinations. Sleep offers neurons that are used while we are awake a chance to briefly shut down and repair themselves. Without sleep, neurons may become so drained of energy that they eventually begin to malfunction. Sleep also gives the brain a chance to exercise important neuronal connections that might otherwise degenerate from lack of activity.

Associated Sleep Disorders

Each year 20 million Americans experience some form of mild sleeping problems, while 40 million Americans suffer from chronic, long-term sleep disorders. These disorders, and the sleep deprivation which occurs, plays havoc with daily life activities. Likewise, they can account for over $16 billion in medical costs each year. Once they are properly diagnosed, the over 70 sleep disorders can be successfully managed. The most common sleep disorders include:

Sleep Apnea is a disorder of interrupted breathing during sleep, while depriving the person of oxygen. The windpipe tends to collapse during breathing while asleep, forcing the person to gasp, snore or snort. This can happen over a hundred times a night. The constant awakenings can leave the patient constantly tired, and may lead to various personality disorders, including depression. Fat buildup, or loss of muscle tone, is usually the contributing factor.

Restless Leg Syndrome (RLS) is a disorder of the nervous system that causes the legs to jerk or uncontrollably move, usually while sleeping. Medications, pregnancy, chronic diseases, and sleep deprivation are some of the many causes. Once correctly diagnosed, RLS can often be successfully treated.

Insomnia is characterized by the inability and/or difficulty in falling asleep, which can result from a plethora of factors, including diet, stress, medications, or chronic health ailments. This tends to increase with age, affecting approximately 30 percent of men and 40 percent of women.

Narcolepsy involves the loss of the brain's ability to regulate sleep/wake cycles normally. People with narcolepsy experience excessive sleepiness; intermittent, uncontrollable episodes of falling asleep during the daytime; hallucinations, Cataplexy (a sudden loss of muscle tone); and/or sleep paralysis.

It's possible to have a sleep disorder if you are excessively tired throughout the day, it takes you more than 30 minutes to fall asleep each night, or when you are awake you feel unrested. If you think you might have a sleep problem, try these steps:

- ***Relax Before Bed*** - A warm bath, reading, or other relaxing routines help make it easier to fall sleep. You can make them part of your bedtime ritual.
- ***Avoid alcohol, nicotine and caffeine*** - Alcohol effects both REM sleep and deep sleep, which makes for a very unsatisfying sleep. Smokers tend to sleep very lightly, and due to nicotine withdrawal, often wake up early in the morning. Sources that contain caffeine, such as non-herbal teas, coffee, diet drugs, pain relievers, soft drinks and chocolate, should be avoided before you retire as they act as a stimulant, keeping you awake.
- ***Set a Schedule*** - Go to bed at a set time each night and get up

at the same time each morning. Disrupting this schedule could lead to insomnia.

- *Sleep Until Sunlight* - If possible, wake up with the sun, or use very bright lights in the morning. Sunlight helps the body's internal biological clock reset itself each day. Sleep experts recommend exposure to an hour of morning sunlight for people having problems falling asleep.
- *Control Bedroom Temperature* - Maintain a comfortable temperature in the bedroom. Extreme temperatures may prevent you from falling asleep, or disrupt your sleep, so keep your temperature at a comfortable level.
- *Exercise* - Try to exercise at least 20 to 30 minutes a day, at least 5 to 6 hours before retiring. Daily exercise often helps people sleep. However, a workout right before bedtime is known to interfere with sleep.
- *Don't Lie Awake In Bed* - If you can't sleep, get up and do something else. Watch some TV, listen to music or read a book until you feel tired.
- *Take a Nap* - Taking a nap can be a great way to increase your sleep, improve your energy, intensify your productivity, and recharge you.

If all else fails:

- **Keep a Sleep Diary:** Track your sleeping patterns and all other behaviors for several days. This may help to make a connection between your sleep quality and your daily activities.
- **Improve Your Sleep Habits:** Make changes, whether small or big, in your sleep habits for a few weeks to see if you can figure out what is causing you to sleep poorly.
- **Find a Sleep Center and Doctor:** If your sleep doesn't improve, take your sleep diary to a sleep center or sleep doctor for further testing.

Proper sleep habits are the key to getting a good night's sleep. Stress, caffeine, alcohol, exercise, and various other factors that I've just discussed can affect the quality and quantity of our sleep. Changing your habits will help you sleep like a baby.

The intelligent Mattress

I was first exposed to the importance of sleep, and the effects of lack of sleep, while I was in college. Of course, I am not referring to the late nights I stayed up studying or stayed out all night partying! I am referring to a class that I took. In the class, we discussed the topics of why we sleep, the stages of sleep, and what is happening in the mind and body while we sleep. It was fascinating and absolutely critical to being healthy and enjoying your life.

Because the class made such an impression on me, I have always discussed how important proper rest is with all my patients. Although there wasn't much I could do at that time, other than recommend a good pillow, I nonetheless gave my patients the best information and sleeping tips that I had. Then one day a young man walked in to my office and asked if I had heard of a company called *Intellibed*. At that time, I had not heard of Intellibed and to be honest, I was not too interested in a mattress company or me, as a physician, selling mattresses to my patients.

However, I did ask if they had any smaller pieces of the intelligel pads for me to be able to give to my friends in wheelchairs.

When I first started my practice, I thought that the best way to meet people was to get involved in my community by doing philanthropic work and giving back. So I started working with the Nevada Special Olympics and was once on the board of Opportunity Village, which is a wonderful organization that provides employment for individuals with mental and physical disabilities. Due to city cutbacks and financial restraints, some programs were either cut down or cut out. As I found that to be sad and unacceptable, I started my own non-profit, which we discussed in the previous chapter - KISMIF. For more information please visit Kismiffundraising.com.

If you have never seen a wheelchair event, I promise you, you will be amazed at the level of play. I work with some amazing individuals that are physically disabled and confined to wheelchairs. They play with the same aggression and intensity as any other professional athlete that I have worked with.

However, there were a few injuries that were more specific to them that I had not prepared myself for, or for that matter even considered treating. Something so small, so harmless, could be so deadly. *Heat or pressure sores* were some of the most prevalent injuries that I was now treating, and that is where the Intellibed comes in to play.

Although pressure sores may sound benign, they actually can be very serious for someone in a wheelchair. Individuals in wheelchairs have to be very careful of the injuries that occur to their paralyzed limbs. A simple heat or pressure sore for a paralyzed person leads to an infection, which then leads to sickness, and sometimes even early death.

As I mentioned, I was not interested in selling mattresses, but I was interested in getting wheelchair pads for my friends in chairs. Because of the "Gel" Intellibeds are made of, it's perfect at preventing pressure or heat sores. The gel creates very little pressure on the legs and spine of the person in the chair, and the Intellibed doesn't hold heat like foam or other kinds of surfaces. This makes the Intellibeds perfect for people in wheelchairs.

Luckily for me, Intellibed agreed to provide me with some wheelchair

Pads, and in return, they asked me to take one of their mattresses home, personally sample the bed, and provide my personal opinion and feedback. It only took about a week, and I was completely sold. Immediately I noticed that I fell asleep quickly, and I stayed asleep the entire night. I woke up fresh and energized, and for the first time in my life, I actually "FELT" how important proper sleep really was. Now going to bed is something that I look forward to. Below is an article written about the Intellibed phenomenon:

> "IntelliGEL®, as it is referred to in the medical field, has been in use in North American hospitals for over a decade. Its non-linear compressibility produces sufficient weight re-distribution to reverse and heal level four pressure sores in long term care settings. Gel technology in the burn unit promotes the healing of third degree burns by maximizing surface blood circulation. In conjunction with medical grade pressure relief, the non-linear compressibility of IntelliGEL® minimizes spinal deflection at the hips and shoulders by re-distributing support along the length of the spine. This re-distribution produces superior spinal alignment that results in a reduction or elimination of back pain. By modifying the compressibility of support layers underneath the IntelliGEL® according to individual needs, an IntelliGEL® mattress supports recovery and stabilizes chronic conditions with superior circulation, sleep posture and sleep quality. IntelliBED is a line of mattresses and related products manufactured by Advance Comfort Technologies, Inc. (ACTI), located in Holladay, Utah. These mattresses are based on intelli-GEL, a honeycombed co-polymer gel developed by EdiZone, also a Utah company. This gel was tested and sold by Gaymar Industries in hospitals and other health care institutions. ACTI developed intelli-GEL products for home use. As of the date of this review, only Advanced Comfort Technologies and intelliBED are licensed to manufacture and sell home bedding products using Intelli-GEL. Currently, IntelliBED has stores in eight

states and two Canadian provinces. IntelliBED mattresses are also prescribed by and sold through participating doctors."

According to Intellibed: *"Most manufacturers are still making mattresses with the same materials used since 1960 – materials that can be harmful, even toxic, to the body. With thorough research, doctor and patient interviews, and extensive third-party testing, we designed and manufactured the mattress the other mattress companies don't want you to know about!*

> *"We own the exclusive rights to the Intelli-GEL® technology patent – the only gel that can sense out and relieve pressure points! intelliBED was founded on the idea that it is possible to perfect the science of sleep. Intelli-GEL sleep surfaces are used in hospitals where they've been proven to be the most effective way to treat serious wound care patients like those suffering from bed sores or burns. These Intelli-GEL-based hospital sleep surfaces cost well over $10,000. We lowered the cost by about 75% by cutting out all the middlemen. Our intelliBEDs, and the Intelli-GEL that goes in them, are manufactured in our Utah factory and are exclusively available to the public through intelliBED or our network of wellness professionals, who help their patients achieve the healing qualities of deep sleep, and the critical role the intelliBED plays in achieving it."*

I now have Intellibeds in my medical center for patients to rest on after treatment or coaching. I personally have an Intellibed in every room of my home, and I recommend the Intellibed mattress to every single patient I see or work with. You can find out more information on the Intellibed mattresses on my website, and I have in place an affiliate Patient Program for my patients to get discounts. Also, if I deem it medically necessary, I can write a prescription to provide a tax person, to establish it as a possible Durable Medical Equipment write-off.

Chapter 13

The Sustainable Power of the Tower

Thomas A. Edison once said: *"The doctor of the future will give no medicine, but will interest her or his patients in the care of the human frame, in a proper diet, and in the cause and prevention of disease."* I believe in that quote, and that is why I have established that philosophy as my foundation to diagnose, treat, and educate my patients about their individual bodies and minds.

We all know that good nutrition is synonymous with good health, and that a well-balanced diet consisting of fruits, vegetables, and good meat sources is the best way to stay healthy. Personally, I prefer a more aggressive diet for those who want to push their physical fitness to an ultra-level. Specifically, I recommend more cholesterol-based animal proteins, because of their nutrient density and bio-availability, such as red meats, whole eggs and whole fat diary. However, vegetables are essential to health, so I provide many different opportunities for my patients to improve the nutritional value of the foods that they eat. The Tower Garden is just one example. If you're a patient of ours, you can come in and take whatever vegetables that we are growing at the time. We have vegetables growing in our office, and if you want them, come get them.

Research has proven that a properly balanced diet and consistent exercise can prevent many diseases such as diabetes, heart disease, and even certain cancers. Let's quickly discuss diabetes as an example. For years the medical community had it all backwards. Instead of using drugs to cure or prevent these diseases, we should be using nutrition and exercises along with the regulation of blood sugars. Most often the medical community uses Metformin, a drug used to treat diabetes. They considered it a successful medicine due to its ability to reduce blood sugars. However, exercise has proven to be twice as effective as Metformin for reducing blood sugars. The important thing to remember is that hitting yourself with carbs every meal will likely continue to keep your blood sugars elevated or spiked. Simply using a drug will not stop the actual disease processes.

Tell me which you would rather have: good food, to feel better and have more energy, or the many side effects of drugs like Metformin? Here are just a few of the nasty side effects associated with Metformin: *Diarrhea, Bloating, Stomach pain, Heartburn, Gas, Indigestion, Constipation, Metallic taste in mouth, Headache, Flush of skin, Nail changes, Muscle pain.* Sound fun?

Although I do not agree with a lot of what the USDA recommends, I do agree that at least one third of your plate should be filled with *good* fruits and/or vegetables. Unfortunately, most people don't abide by that rule and do not even eat one meal a day consisting of fruits or veggies. The ramifications of not having a healthy diet is always disease.

The sad truth is that the vegetables we purchase from our local grocery stores are not fresh and often even on the verge of spoilage. Even though the produce may look fresh, sometimes it is days or weeks old, has been sprayed with pesticides and herbicides, and is totally deficient in any true nutritional value. Who wants to eat old, bland, sickly produce?

Personally, I love fruits and vegetables. A bite of cold watermelon is wonderful on a hot summer's day. Routinely, vegetables are a part of every meal that I have. Even when I travel, I always make sure that vegetables are incorporated into my daily diet. Here's an interesting fact and more to what I am talking about in regards to thinking outside the box: Did you know that most of the produce for the restaurants in the Chicago's O'Hare Airport comes from what they actually grow *inside* the airport? There is a collection of tower gardens (or the like) inside the airport that the restaurants use to feed the many travelers, and they do not even know it. If one can do it, why can't they all do it?

Now that's Self-Sustainable!

To make sure that I always get the freshest vegetables, I have a Tower Garden® in my medical facility. I actually grow vegetables right there in my office. Not only do I use the produce for myself and my staff, but I also give the produce to my patients for free.

So what is a Tower Garden®? It's basically a vertical growing system which uses an air or mist environment, as opposed to a soil environment. Imagine being able to grow your own vegetables on the 36th floor patio of a New York hi-rise or in your kitchen in North Dakota in January. Anyone can do it and almost anywhere.

Because My Tower Garden® is in my office and it has become so popular, our patients now want to learn how they can purchase one to use in their own homes and offices. Once our patients have had a food sensitivity test, and we determine the proper diet for each individual patient, we then teach them which foods they should be growing and which foods they should stay away from.

To help our patients get on the right path, we teach them about growing food at home, as well as the proper lighting and watering to maximize their harvests. After I get my patients out of pain, we get their body chemistry right, I get them losing weight and feeling better. The end result is to offer them self-sustainable options to implement into their daily lives. We educate them on many other aspects of how to become self-sustainable and able to be self-correcting and self-motivated. They don't have to do it all, but it's available to them if they want it.

That's where the self-sustainable aspect comes into play. Ultimately we make sure that if you have any food sensitivities, or you have any particular type of problem that is causing inflammation in the body, we'll help you remove those from your diet and oftentimes from your surroundings. So everything that you put into your body would ultimately be suited for your body, as opposed to the laundry list of vitamins, minerals, and other bogus things that are out there designed to only make money for the people selling them. Everything we recommend, suggest, or offer for you is catered and structured for your body - your protein powders, your foods in your diet, great recipes, and functional exercises. Everything is catered towards what your body wants and needs. We'll go into more detail on that subject in a later chapter. Ultimately, I encourage my patients to take this education and expand upon it. I start by

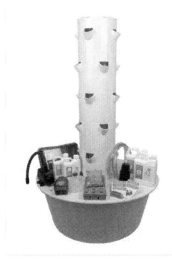

saying, "If you use a tower garden, you could grow your own vegetables at home, save money, and maybe even save your life. Here's how. It's simple, cheap, and easy." I get them to become self-sustainable from a dietary standpoint first, and then I get them to become more self-sustainable in other areas of their lives like solar, wind, water, composting, and other self-sustainable opportunities.

Tower Power

The Tower Garden Growing System® was originally developed by Tim Blank, who founded *Future Growing* (www.futuregrowing.com) because he had a dream that "someday everybody on the planet would have access to healthy food in their own home and local community." His patented 5-foot vertical garden comes with everything you need to grow healthy herbs, fruits and vegetables, either indoors or out, all year long.

The nice thing about using this system is that you literally don't need any gardening experience. It's easy to use for people of all ages – from children to adults to senior citizens. It has a compact, state-of-the-art, vertical system which easily fits into your lifestyle on your rooftop, terrace or patio. However, the best part is that it fits into your healthy diet.

Some of the benefits of the Tower Garden include:

1) **It's Healthy** - There's no pesticides or herbicides used.
2) **It's Convenient** - No need to run to the store when you want fresh tomatoes for your salad or melons for breakfast.
3) **It's Easy** – No weeds, pests or soil to worry about. It's easy to assemble and maintain, and fits relatively anywhere.
4) **It Produces More** – 30% more produce than soil-based.
5) **It Tastes Better** – Fresh always tastes better, therefore, you eat more.
6) **Cost Effective** – No need to spend money on unnecessary products and tools needed for traditional gardens.
7) **Cost per Unit** - One head of cauliflower costs $3.45 at the store. One head grown at home costs pennies.
8) **It's Quicker** - Can produce crops in less time than it takes to grow in soil.
9) **Better Environment** - Recycles 100% of its nutrients and water.
10) **No Gardening Experience Needed** – People love to feel a sense of accomplishment.

Chapter 14

Kicking the Crap Out of Your Kitchen

There are so many changes when it comes to nutrition or diet. It seems that every other day you hear something different from what you heard the day before. If you eat too much salt, it is the worst thing you could ever do, and then the next day you read that salt will save your life. Because of all of the inconsistencies and confusion, I work closely with a nutritionist. A **nutritionist** is a person who advises on matters of food and nutrition and how that impacts your health. Different professional names are used — some examples include: nutrition scientist, public health nutritionist, dietitian-nutritionist, clinical nutritionist, and sports nutritionist. The individuals we work with are the very best at customizing a diet based upon science and formal interviews with our patients. I advise all my patients to have an initial work-up by a trained specialist. They will be able to provide invaluable information and resources, as well great tasting recipes.

Make these flavorful foods at home and you can save money while eating healthy and responsibly:

Bread - You can purchase a versatile bread machine, or simply make healthy and incredible tasting bread varieties in cooking tins in your oven. The list of healthy ingredients you can incorporate into homemade bread, like whole grains and fruits, is virtually endless.

Tomato-based products - When you make your own pasta sauce, ketchup and salsa, you dictate exactly what healthy ingredients you are using. When you purchase these tomato-based items at a grocery store, they have likely gone through an extreme manufacturing process.

Soup - Store-bought soup is notoriously high in sodium. If you are like me, crunched for time, you can slow cook several servings of healthy, tasty, homemade soup in a slow cooker and freeze for instant enjoyment later.

Sauces and dressings - There are also dozens, if not hundreds, of great tasting dressings and sauces you can make right at home using healthy ingredients. This also means never purchasing expensive, processed sauces or dressings again.

Yogurt - Do-it-yourself yogurt is so much healthier than the products offered at your favorite supermarket. Some yogurt can be healthy off-the-shelf, but most of it is extremely processed.

Guacamole - This is another "made at home," processed food alternative which is not only healthier when you create it in your own kitchen, but also less expensive than the store-bought variety.

Granola and energy bars - There are multiple healthy recipes online for making your own granola bars. The same goes for energy boosting bars, which you can make for up to 50% less money than purchasing the unhealthy, processed options at your supermarket.

Dealing With Processed Foods Cravings

One of the best ways to deal with an addiction is to remove its physical presence - clean out your pantry and remove processed foods from your living environment. After all, if a sugar-filled snack or processed microwave meal is not available, you can't eat it.

But sometimes you may experience cravings for processed foods when you are away from home. A great way to kill those desires is to keep healthy and delicious tasting fruits, vegetables, homemade granola bars, and other unprocessed snacks in your car and workplace.

Studies have shown that just drinking 8 to 16 ounces of water can fight a food craving for more than an hour. Also, if you eat 5 or 6 meals throughout the day, your stomach constantly stays full. This means less of a chance that you will give in to the urges created by a processed food that is calling your name.

Keeping a food journal is also helpful here. Whenever you experience a craving for unhealthy, processed food, write down your feelings. Then look at what happened just before the craving hit. Did you receive an exceptionally good or bad piece of news? Emotional eating is not in response to true hunger, and is often attached to a sugar addiction, which can be a problem with processed foods.

Surrounding yourself with like-minded individuals is extremely important. If you have someone you can talk to that is also trying to steer clear of the dangers of processed foods, your chances of eating smart and never giving into unhealthy cravings are much higher.

You should also keep a "Why?" belief statement on you at all times. This can be simply a small card that fits in your wallet, pocket or purse. Write down the reasons why you are avoiding processed foods and trying to eat a much healthier diet. This can provide the motivation to beat even the strongest cravings.

Eating healthy means avoiding heavily processed foods. You can actually save money by treating your body to a much healthier diet in many cases. There are cookbooks, DVDs, courses and web videos, which arm you with the proper information regarding processed foods and their dangers, and how to avoid them.

And the information included in this book acts as a primer to get you started on a path towards healthy and smart eating. So, formulate a game plan for eating a clean, whole, plant-based diet beginning today, and you will treat yourself to a happier and healthier tomorrow.

Chapter 15

Fine Tuning Your Diet

As we age, it's even advisable to eat FEWER daily meals and to avoid carbs when you anticipate a sedentary period following a meal. The fewer meals (3 a day on light training days and 4 a day on heavy training days) will allow the body to remain sensitive to insulin, which will improve and speed up glucose absorption, thereby causing blood sugars not to stay elevated longer than necessary. Eating carbs post workout is ideal, but, at the risk of over emphasizing the importance of something like carb timing, just reducing the frequency at which carbs are consumed, not even the quantity, could be very beneficial for reducing HA1C levels. This is contrary to the conventional wisdom that 5 small meals or "grazing" is better for dieting, but it's consistent with the research that supports your calorie equation (In - Out) whether those calories are consumed in 3 meals or 6. Only the psychological hunger factor is really to be considered, when determining the number of meals in order to prevent people from binging, but there are two schools of thought there as well.

There are some things I would like you to consider to help stay healthy:

1. Fat-free dairy is high in sugar, relative to its fat and protein content. Whether or not carbs in general should be consumed at every meal should be carefully monitored because it can lead to insulin resistance and elevated HA1C levels. I mention this particularly because I believe that high insulin levels and prolonged periods of elevated blood sugars are the primary culprit for aging and many health-related problems.

2. Processed vegetable oils, such as canola are nothing short of poison. Cold pressed oils such as extra Virgin Olive oil and Coconut oil are good, but there's no need to overemphasize the value of Fish Oils in general,

particularly not at the sacrifice of a little bit of grass fed red meat, which brings me to my next suggestion:

3. Grass fed red meat in the diet is packed with highly bio-available heme-iron, creatine, B vitamins, zinc, magnesium, etc. I believe some healthy cholesterol in the diet has beneficial effects for the brain and possibly in delaying Alzheimer's. However, I do think that the improvement in HDL cholesterol is more a result of reducing H1C levels than consuming healthy cholesterol.

4. I'm not a fan of soy.

5. I'm not a fan of icing or anti-inflammatories (NSAIDS). It's much better to use compression and active recovery.

Chapter 16

Clean Eating For Busy People

Everywhere you turn you hear about the dangers of processed food. Everyone is telling you to eat more fruits and vegetables and to avoid "processed foods." But what exactly is processed food? Just about anyone can look at a chicken nugget and realize that whatever chicken might be present has gone through an extreme modification.

By definition, processed food is food that has been altered from its natural state. So, a package of chopped lettuce is actually processed. It has been made more convenient and then bagged. Those types of processed foods are usually good for you. The types of manufactured foods you want to avoid are those that involve combining raw ingredients and chemicals into food-like items.

Some foods that qualify for the definition of processed are actually improved. Some milk, juices and other beverages have vitamins added to them to make them healthier. But for the most part, processed foods should be avoided because a lot of the process that gets them from nature to your table includes packing them with preservatives, sugar and trans fats.

Pesticides can also be a part of the process. When foods are being grown, they are often treated with chemicals to ward off hungry bugs and insects. That is why eating clean or organic foods can cut down on the amount of toxins a human being consumes every day by as much as 80%, according to the Environmental Working Group.

When ingredients such as sugar, fat and salt are added to food to enhance flavor, or make it last longer, this type of processed product can end up getting more than the recommended amounts of those items into your body. Health hazards and addictions to salt and sugar are often the result.

Those types of items are also usually higher in calories, which means packing on the pounds. And if you eat a lot of red meat that has been processed, you run a much higher risk of contracting certain forms of cancer. So you want to avoid products that have lost nutrients and gained unhealthy and unneeded chemicals and alternatives.

Just how can you spot which food is good for you and which is unhealthy? You need to learn how to spot "clean" foods.

Identifying "Clean" Foods

You may have heard people talk about eating a "clean" diet. While there is no specific definition for clean foods, eating clean means sticking with foods that are as close as possible to their natural state. You want to avoid preservatives, coloring, and man-made chemicals.

Drinking a lot of water aids a clean diet by keeping your system flushed. For the most part, you want to target fruits, vegetables, whole foods (items that have been processed or refined as little as possible and are free from additives or other artificial substances) and a plant-based diet.

So how do you identify clean foods? When reading food labels, which you should be doing all the time, you want to avoid most foods with more than 5 ingredients.

One-ingredient foods, such as apples, oranges and other fruit in their natural state, are examples of clean foods. And you definitely want to avoid the big 3 added ingredients which cause the most havoc to your health - salt, sugar and dietary fats.

Another healthy tip is to turn away from those products that are "made with "whole grains." Instead, go for 100% whole-grain products. Refined grains, such as bread, cereal and pasta, which are made from white flour, should also be avoided. But whole-grain pasta, cereal and bread are considered clean foods.

Generally speaking, if a food item has just one ingredient or is as close to its natural state as possible, it qualifies for clean eating. This means no more cans of soup, candy bars, fried chicken and French fries. Fresh poultry, seafood and meat are usually fine, as long as you take it easy on the creams or sauces.

You can follow these tips for spotting clean foods:

1. If you read a food label and there are ingredients with names that you cannot pronounce, put it back on the shelf.
2. If you see the following ingredients, you are looking at extremely processed foods – corn syrup, fruit juice concentrate, maltose, cane sugar, sodium, partially hydrogenated vegetable oil.
3. If the food you are thinking about purchasing is in a package, it has been processed to some point.
4. If there are more than 5 ingredients, look for an alternative.
5. Avoid trans fats, monosodium glutamate (MSG), high fructose corn syrup, other sugars, sodium and other salts, and white flour.
6. Most foods with organic labels are cleaner than other options.
7. And if you purchase any of the following Dirty Dozen foods, choose organic whenever you can, and wash thoroughly before eating.

The Dirty Dozen foods are so named by the Environmental Working Group because they are extremely high in man-made chemicals and pesticides. When grown in the traditional manner, these 12 foods tested positive for anywhere from 47 to 67 different chemicals:

- Apples
- Sweet bell peppers
- Cherries
- Imported grapes
- Celery
- Strawberries
- Domestic blueberries
- Nectarines
- Kale, spinach and collard greens
- Potatoes
- Lettuce
- Peaches

Now that you know how to spot clean foods, let's take a look at the best reasons for steering clear of processed foods.

Eight Top Reasons to Cut Out Processed Foods

You know that a diet rich in fresh fruits, vegetables and whole grains is healthy for you. But do you know exactly why you should be cutting processed foods out of your life? Let's take a look at the top 8 reasons for steering clear of processed foods:

1. *They can be full of high fructose corn syrup*
   Why is high fructose corn syrup (HFCS) so dangerous to your health? Because it contributes to liver deterioration, plaque buildup in your blood vessels, has been shown to cause diabetes, it accelerates the natural aging process in your body and can contain unhealthy mercury poisons. And, it is used in more and more processed food products all the time.

2. *Many of them include monosodium glutamate*

MSG, or monosodium glutamate, is a form of salt which has been chemically changed to enhance the flavor of many popular processed foods. It has been directly linked to weight gain and obesity, and negatively affects how full you feel when you are eating. This can lead to binge eating, since your brain never knows when you are full.

Liver inflammation, kidney failure, and even brain damage are possible byproducts of heavy exposure to MSG. Unfortunately, it is the world's most popular flavor enhancer. And it can be listed under any of the following names – acid hydrolyzed vegetable protein, hydrolyzed corn, MSG, plant protein extract, yeast extract, plus others.

3. *Low-fat often means high in sugar*

Many processed and manufactured foods boast about being low-fat or no-fat in nature. The process which pulls fat out of those foods also involves adding HFCS, sucrose, lactose and glucose, as well as other yummy tasting but unhealthy sweeteners.

Sugar triggers the "feel good" transmitters in your brain, and this can cause an addiction to sweet tasting, processed foods. Sugar can have a devastating effect on your health, and is believed by many doctors and nutritionists to be the leading cause of chronic disease and obesity in today's modern societies.

4. *Important nutrients are processed out*

Many processed foods are created to last longer on the shelf, and taste better than when they existed in their natural state. This oftentimes involves removing wonderful phytonutrients, vitamins and minerals, either intentionally or indirectly.

By its very definition, processing foods leads to a non-natural state. So many of the healthy components that nature packs into its foods are lacking when that food is processed.

5. *Unnatural and dangerous chemicals are added*
We just mentioned that food manufacturers are usually only interested in creating products that last as long as possible, are inexpensive to make, and taste great so you continue to buy them. How do they do this? In laboratories they find chemicals, like fructose, that trigger an addictive response in your brain.

They then inject those chemicals into foods during the manufacturing and packaging processes. This unneeded MSG, sugar, salt, and a long list of man-made chemicals finds its way into processed food, which is unhealthy at best and dangerous at worst.

6. *Clean foods are easier on your digestive system*
We just discussed how cheap, flavor enhancing, unhealthy chemicals get into your processed food. Your body identifies these as poisons and toxins, and works very hard to rid your system of them. But they are much harder to digest than the foods which nature intended men and women to eat. This makes your digestive tract work harder than it has to, and this can lead to a long list of gastrointestinal problems and health issues.

7. *Whole foods are less expensive than their processed counterparts*
Junk food addicts often claim that eating healthy foods is just too expensive. But several studies, like one published by the Rodale Institute, show that the opposite is actually true. For instance, they show that one serving of 100% organic chili (made with fresh ingredients) costs roughly $0.50 less than a can of microwavable chili like you would normally purchase at

the grocery store.

8. ***You will begin to feel healthier almost immediately***
    Processed foods contain a lot of junk your body does not need. This can include phosphates which actually weaken your bones and organs. The excess sugar in processed foods can lead to weight gain and heart problems, and many manufactured foods can lead to chronic inflammation, dementia, respiratory failure and multiple neurologic problems. When you eat clean and avoid processed food, you become healthier.

Processed Food Alternatives

You might be thinking that you won't have the time to purchase and prepare whole foods and healthy fruits, vegetables and grains. After all, your life is very busy already. But you can benefit from a plant-based and clean eating diet without making your lifestyle more hectic than it already is. Just follow these processed food alternative tips for eating clean and smart, and you may actually find that your healthier eating habits save you more time and energy than your processed food past.

Forming a game plan, centered on healthy eating, is essential if you are going to avoid processed foods and the dangers they can deliver. Sit down and create a realistic shopping, cooking, and food storage plan that includes the following 4 tips:

1. ***Clean out your pantry***
    Check the labels on all of the food you currently have in your home. Pull out everything that lists MSG, HFCS, added sugar, excess salt and white flour. If you feel that throwing away this food is a waste of money, donate it to your local homeless shelter. However, you are definitely going to have to rid your home of addictive and unhealthy processed food temptations to begin the clean eating process.

2. *Prepare and cook multiple meals at once*

   Batch cooking makes sense for a lot of reasons. When you purchase, prepare and then cook multiple meals at once, you can often benefit from lower prices by buying larger quantities. Whatever mess you make in the kitchen only has to be dealt with at one time. Also, by packaging, preparing, cooking and storing several meals at a time, rather than single meals several times a week, you minimize your time investment.

3. *Get the whole family involved*

   You are busy. So is everyone else in your family. Why not schedule a couple of hours every week so the entire family can help out in your shopping, preparing and batch cooking processes? Not only will this save time and money in the long run, but it will also instill important and healthy eating habits in your children.

4. *Take a road trip*

   Do some research and find out where the whole food markets, bazaars and shops are in your area. You may be surprised to find that natural, locally grown foods, free of pesticides, fertilizers and chemicals, are just around the corner, and less expensive than the ones you have been buying in the supermarket.

Avoiding Processed Food When Dining Out

Once you begin to avoid processed food, you will find yourself eating out less frequently. But there are always going to be times when seasonal holidays, birthday celebrations, and get-togethers with family and friends, make it tough for you to eat in a healthy manner.

However, there are some steps you can take which will help you avoid processed food any time you eat away from your home. For instance, avoid processed salad dressings. Instead, choose oil and vinegar the next time you join your friends for dinner, either in their home or a restaurant.

Choose grilled over fried as an option whenever possible. Food items, which are processed and prepackaged, may be fried in oil that contains trans fats. When eating at a restaurant, don't be afraid to ask your chef or waiter how certain meals are prepared.

Another great way of avoiding processed foods when you eat out is to take advantage of the growing movement towards healthy dining options. Many restaurant menus contain gluten-free, heart-healthy and non-processed sections, making avoiding processed foods easy. Sometimes these are not printed, but all you have to do is ask, and you might get a meal prepared in a healthier way.

You might want to skip dessert as well. Desserts are notoriously high in sugar and other processed additives, which serve no other reason than to preserve them longer and get you hooked on their taste.

One of the best ways to keep from eating unhealthy, manufactured foods when attending a party or gathering is to bring your own dish. Whether at a friend's house or restaurant, skip flavored beverages and stick with water.

You can also eat a small portion of something healthy and filling before you head out, so you limit the number of processed calories you consume.

Eat Wild Game

It used to be that most people grew up eating wild game; however, that is a very rare thing these days. Now, there is ample evidence of the healthy benefits of eating wild game. It is even becoming fashionable, which is a rare thing these days, with many restaurants now offering wild game as prized menu items. Game meat is leaner than meat from domesticated animals, and the fat on game meat may have a slightly stronger, earthier taste, and should be removed before cooking. Because game meat is so lean, it is best to cook it slowly – either braise in liquid, or roast and baste frequently to make sure it is tender.

The following is the nutritional value of a variety of game meats compared with beef or pork.

Nutritional value of game meat (3ounces)	Calories	Fat (grams)	Saturated fat (grams)	Cholesterol (mgs)
Deer	134	3	1	85
Elk	124	2	1	62
Moose	114	1	Trace	66
Caribou	142	4	1	93
Antelope	127	2	1	107
Beef	259	18	7	75
Pork	214	13	5	73

*Composite of all cuts, trimmed and roasted. Source: USDA Nutrient Data Laboratory

The nutritional value and quality of the meat depends on:

- Type of animal - deer, elk, moose, caribou, or antelope.
- Age of the animal - Younger animals are usually more tender.
- Sex of the animal – Usually the males have more testosterone and other musk hormones that create a gamier flavor.
- Diet of the animal – What the animal eats plays a huge role in flavor. Animals with access to abundant food sources tend to have more body fat, so their meat is higher in fat and calories.

Some game meat is higher in dietary cholesterol than domestic meats, but the combination of more lean body tissue, generally fewer calories, less saturated fat, and significantly higher percentage of cholesterol-reducing, polyunsaturated fatty acids makes game a heart-healthy choice.

Game meat also has a significantly higher content of EPA (Eicosapentaenoic Acid, a type of omega 3 fatty acid, which is a good type of oil, often referred to as fish oil) than domestic meat. EPA is thought to reduce the risk of developing atherosclerosis, one of the major causes of heart attack and stroke. Game meat is usually higher in iron and is extremely nutrient dense.

Wild game contains more than five times the amount of polyunsaturated fat per gram than is found in domestic livestock, according to Dr. S. Boyd Eaton of the Emory University School of Medicine. About four percent of wild game fat is polyunsaturated, whereas domestic beef has an undetectable or minimal amount. Recent studies have shown that polyunsaturated fats (or "good" Cholesterol) – are actually beneficial, and offset the negative impacts of saturated fats (or bad cholesterol). The virtues of game meat are especially important to people with specific health conditions, including heart disease or kidney failure.

What I Recommend To Eat

I don't mean to be nit-picky, but I think there are some persistent myths that have arisen from the government's erroneous war on fats and their over-emphasis on carbohydrates in the food pyramid. However, on the next page are lists of foods, spices, and other food sources that I highly recommend, in addition to cholesterol based animal proteins such as red meats, whole eggs and whole fat diary:

VEGETABLES

- Amaranth greens – a variety of Spinach
- Avocado
- Bell Peppers
- Chayote (Mexican Squash)
- Cucumber
- Dandelion greens
- Garbanzo beans
- Green bananas
- Izote – cactus flower – naturally grows in the southwest
- Kale
- Lettuce (No Iceberg)
- Mushrooms (No Shiitake)
- Mexican Cactus
- Okra
- Olives
- Onions
- Squash
- Tomato – cherry and/or plum
- Tomatillo
- Turnip greens
- Watercress
- Zucchini

FRUITS

- Apples
- Bananas – (original banana)
- Berries – (no cranberries)
- Cantaloupe
- Cherries
- Coconuts
- Currants
- Elderberries
- Dates
- Figs
- Grapes- (with seeds)

- Limes (key limes)
- Mango
- Melons- seeded
- Oranges (Seville or sour preferred)
- Papayas
- Peaches
- Pears
- Plums
- Prickly Pear or Cactus Fruit
- Prunes
- Raisins – (with seeds)

HERBAL TEAS
- Allspice
- Anise
- Burdock
- Chamomile
- Elderberry
- Fennel
- Ginger
- Raspberry

SPICES AND SEASONINGS
- Basil
- Bay leaf
- Cloves
- Dill
- Oregano
- Parsley
- Savory

PUNGENT AND SPICY FLAVORS
- Achiote
- Cayenne
- Cilantro
- Coriander
- Habanero

SALTY FLAVORS
- Pure Sea Salt (Himalayan Sea Salt)
- Powdered Granulated Seaweed (Kelp/Dulce/Nori – has "sea taste")

SWEET FLAVORS
- 100% Pure Agave Syrup – (from Agave cactus)
- Date Sugar

GRAINS
- Amaranth
- Quinoa
- Rye
- Spelt
- Wild Rice

NUTS AND SEEDS
- Hemp Seed
- Sesame Seeds
- Walnuts
- Brazil Nuts
- Pine Nuts

OILS
- Olive Oil (Do not cook)
- Coconut Oil (Do not cook)
- Grapeseed Oil
- Sesame Oil
- Hempseed Oil
- Avocado Oil

Chapter 17

Living A Sustainable Life

You recycle. You buy organic foods, whenever possible, and you try to combine your errands so you don't use too much fuel. Maybe you carpool to work and occasionally buy and sell from consignment stores. Sustainability is on your radar. You want to be a responsible citizen that takes care of the planet and does what you can to live an environmentally-friendly lifestyle.

When it comes to sustainability, there is a balance. Most people want to do more to live an eco-friendly life, but they also want to make sure that it doesn't consume all of their time, energy, and money.

For example, there's a difference between starting a garden and converting your entire household energy to solar power. One requires a few hours a week of your time, and the other may require several months of renovations and a change in energy consumption that you may not be prepared for.

So how do you know where that balance is? How do you know if you're doing as much as you can do without dramatically changing the way you live your life?

Are You Ready to Take Sustainability to the Next Level?

Sustainability is a lifestyle. As you take steps to live a greener life, you'll make changes to your lifestyle. Are you ready for some changes? Let's take a look at a few questions. The answers will guide you to your next steps:

How Organized Are You?

Do you find that you often create systems to organize your life, your space, and your routine? For example, do you occasionally re-organize the pantry or create chore charts for yourself or your children? If you're often creating systems, that means you're fully capable of tackling a more sustainable life. You might even have what it takes to take on a larger project or lifestyle change.

Are You Ready for a Change?

Change is good. It keeps you fresh. It challenges your mindset and your mental processes. It helps you grow. Adopting a new sustainability project, habit, or system requires a willingness to change. If you feel like you're ready for change and can get excited about it, then you're ready to take sustainability to the next level.

Are You Looking to Feel More Fulfilled, Rewarded, and Engaged?

Living a sustainable lifestyle is rewarding. Sure, some projects are hard work, but that hard work pays off. You'll feel more engaged in life and in your community. You'll also enjoy a feeling of satisfaction when you know that your new habits do have a positive impact on the world.

If you answered yes to any of these questions, then you're ready to take sustainability to the next level. Don't worry; you don't have to go off the grid if you don't want to. Here are eight different ideas to add more sustainable habits and projects to your life. Choose one or all eight - it's up to you:

Self-Sustainability Idea #1 - Fun Ways to Give Back, Live Sustainably, and Enjoy a Simpler Lifestyle

For many, part of living sustainably is creating a sense of community. It's not just a lifestyle; it's a movement. It's a collective approach to make the world a better place and that doesn't just stop with environmental steps. It can include other methods of working with others. Let's take a look at three fun ways to give back, live sustainable and enjoy a simpler lifestyle:

Join a CSA - CSA stands for Community Supported Agriculture.

Basically, CSA members buy shares of a farm and receive the benefits. When you buy a share, the benefits include whatever the farm produces. Some farms focus solely on growing produce. You'll receive weekly bundles of lettuce, onions, and tomatoes in the summer months, and squash and dark leafy greens in the fall. Other farms might sell shares of the livestock they have on the farm. You might get eggs from chickens, milk from goats, or meat from a cow at the end of the year. Some farms sell partial shares, which are good for small families. Whole shares might provide enough weekly produce to feed a large family or multiple families. CSAs are fun because it creates a community. Everyone is welcomed to pitch in at the farm, though you don't have to. You create a routine of visiting the farm and picking up your fresh organic produce. They're great for the local economy and excellent for the environment as most CSAs are organic farms. Additionally, you're not buying produce that had to be shipped from another country to your supermarket, so you're cutting back on your carbon footprint.

- **Join a Food Co-Op** - A food co-op, or cooperative, is an organized grocery store. Members help decide what items are carried in the store and where they come from. In exchange, they also get reduced prices. Most often, items in the market come from local farmers and local companies. You have the ability to buy materials in bulk and to save money. Co-operatives can be fun because you're part of a community of decision makers. It's a lifestyle that many people enjoy.

- **Grow a Community Garden** - Another option to enjoy a simpler lifestyle while giving back is to participate or start a community garden. This type of initiative works well in suburban or urban environments where green space may be limited. Find a plot of land, get permission from the city, and then invite others to participate in the tending of the garden. Those who help out and give their time are able to enjoy the fruits of their labors. It's also a great way to get children involved in the growing process and to help them understand how plants grow and how food is produced.

Finally, if all of these ideas are a bit too time-consuming, or they're unavailable in your area, consider creating a weekly outing to your local farmer's market. You can enjoy the time outside with your friends and family and support local farmers at the same time. And you just can't beat the flavor and nutrition of locally-grown produce.

The next idea takes a look at how to reduce food waste. You'll not only help create a better environment, you'll save money too.

Self- Sustainability Idea #2 - Embracing Alternative Energy

One way to make a huge impact on your energy bill and on the environment is to begin using alternative energy in your home. Some states may still offer tax credit for installing alternative energy systems.

Step One: Choose Your Approach

There are several different alternative energy sources to consider. The most popular are solar and wind. Solar is generally considered the easiest option and the most affordable. Most experts agree that solar panels and systems have never been cheaper.

Fully installed, your solar array might cost around $3 per watt. The average four kilowatt system then costs around $12,000 for the entire system. However, that doesn't include tax credits and the savings. Over 20 years, experts predict the average family could save around $20,000.

Wind and hydro systems are another option. However, they are generally more expensive and more difficult to maintain. Solar is durable and lasts for decades with minimal maintenance.

Step Two: Identify Your Budget and Goals

Decide what you want to accomplish from your alternative energy. For example, if you simply want to recharge your devices without having to plug in, you can invest in small solar charging appliances. If you want to go completely independent and create all your own power, you'll want to take the next step.

Step Three: Get Quotes and Price It Out

There are two general approaches. You can reach out to local installation companies, who can give you the full package. This often includes connecting you to the grid so you can earn energy credits. Or you can install your system yourself.

Step Four: Install and Enjoy

Get your system installed and create a plan to maintain it. Now you can enjoy the fruits of your labor for decades. For fun, track your monthly savings by comparing your new energy bill to last years.

Self- Sustainability Idea #3 - The Lowdown on LED

This sustainability idea is a super easy one. However, the initial financial output may be more than you'd like to take on. We're talking about switching all of your home's light bulbs to LED bulbs.

Why Switch?

According to the EPA, the Environmental Protection Agency, if every household in the United States replaced just one standard incandescent light bulb with an energy-efficient one, the nation would save about $600 million in annual energy costs. That's enough to power three million homes for a year.

You might also be surprised to learn that lighting your home typically accounts for about 20-30 percent of your electric bill. If you have a $50 monthly electric bill, that's a savings of about $150 annually.

Are LED Bulbs Expensive?

The truth is that when compared to a 99 cent, incandescent light bulb, a $25 bulb may seem outrageous. However, here's the thing. That $25 bulb will last twenty years or more, which brings it down to about a dollar a bulb annually.

That incandescent bulb that you buy will probably need to be replaced in four to six months. So, you're actually spending a bit more annually on incandescent bulbs than on LED, but it's negligible. The real savings is in the annual energy savings.

A Strategic Approach

If you're not excited about spending a thousand dollars or more replacing every single light bulb in your home, then you might enjoy this frugal strategy:

Step One: Identify your priority lights

What lights do you use the most? Chances are they're in your kitchen and living room. This is where you spend the most time each day and where the lights are on more. Replace these lights first.

Step Two: Buy in bulk

In many cases, you'll be able to save a bit on LED bulbs if you buy them in multipacks. Make sure you're buying the right size bulb for your fixture. Make the appropriate lumens to watts conversion (there's usually a conversion printed on the packaging).

Look also for the appropriate size base. For example, some lights have pins at the base and others have screw bottoms. Also choose the right size and shape bulb. There's nothing more frustrating than getting a bulb home and realizing it peeks out above your light shade. It's unattractive and irritating.

Step Three: Keep an eye out for sales and coupons

Make a list of the next priority room and keep an eye out for sales and coupons. More and more stores, including your local supermarket, carry LED bulbs, so you should be able to find some savings.

LED bulbs are a simple way to live a more sustainable life. Add them to your home in a way that makes the most financial sense for you.

Self- Sustainability Idea #4 - Reducing Your Food Waste

You might be surprised to learn that, in the United States, more than 34 million tons of food goes to waste on an annual basis. That accounts for around 14 percent of the total waste. The vast majority of this garbage goes into landfills, where it decomposes and creates greenhouse gases. The U.S. Department of Agriculture estimates that people in the U.S. waste about 27 percent of their food.

So what can you do to reduce your food waste? Keep in mind that by reducing the amount of food you throw away, you're actually saving money, too. The following tips and lifestyle changes will help you make sure very little goes to waste:

- Meal Planning - Sit down once or twice a week and plan your meals. Plan what you need for breakfasts, lunches and dinners. Create a list and then shop from the list. Buy only what you need. When you're making the list, keep the recipes in front of you, so you can make sure you buy the right quantity. For example, if the stir fry recipe calls for 10 ounces of chicken, you can buy only around 10 ounces.
- Learn to Love Leftovers - Much of the food that goes to waste in your home is probably due to leftovers. Either change your meal planning so you don't have leftovers, or learn to love them. For example, leftover stir fry may not sound like a typical

breakfast, but it can be quite satisfying. Or, use them for your pack lunch.

- Learn to Preserve or Can Foods - There are many different opportunities to preserve your produce before it goes bad. For example, if you buy an abundance of apples and can't eat them all before they go bad, you can chop them up and freeze them. You can place them in a food dehydrator, or a low temperature oven, and make dried apple slices. You can also cook them down, toss them in a food processor, and make applesauce or apple butter. Or, you can "*CAN*" those extra tomatoes to make sauces or soups.

Finally, if you just can't do anything with that food and it's going to end up in a landfill, consider composting. Composting turns your food scraps and paper scraps into rich soil that you can use in your garden, landscaping or even in your indoor plants. It's a smart way to help keep waste out of landfills and to reduce your food waste.

Self-Sustainability Idea #5 - Composting

What do you do with your vegetable scraps? What about your banana peels, coffee grounds, or egg shells? Whether you have a garden or not, you can turn that everyday kitchen garbage into compost.

Compost is nature's recycling program. Materials decompose and turn into extremely fertile and rich soil. You can use the compost around your outdoor plants, in your houseplants, and of course, you can add it to your lawn or garden. While adding composting to your lifestyle does require adopting a few new habits, it's actually pretty easy to incorporate into the way you live using the following steps:

Step One: Your Containers

You'll need two containers. You'll need a composting bin or area outside. You'll also need something to store your kitchen waste in.

Outdoors, there are different types of bins to consider. Some have a handle on them so you can turn the bin and mix your compost. Others allow you to pop off the top. You mix by hand using a rake or shovel.

Indoors, you want to choose a ceramic or stainless steel container. You'll want it to have a lid.

Step Two: Start Your Compost

Outside, you'll want to position your compost bin in an area where it will be out of your way but convenient. Start your compost with a layer of brown material. Brown material is anything that is dry like twigs, dry leaves, straw, or dried grass. You'll want this material to be a few inches thick. Inside, you can start collecting your kitchen waste.

In general, don't compost any meat, grease, or material that has animal waste on it. You can compost cardboard, fruits and vegetables, egg shells, coffee and tea grounds, and newspapers. If you aren't sure, play it safe and don't add it to your compost.

A word of warning: if you add seeds to your compost, for example apple or tomato seeds, don't be surprised to find plants growing in your compost, or later in your yard where you've placed the compost.

When your indoor container is full, add it to your outdoor compost bin and mix it up.

Step Three: Evaluate and Maintain

Your compost needs to stay moist but not soaking. If it gets too wet, it will mold. If it's too dry, nothing will happen. You can add water to your compost if it's looking dry. Stir your compost every couple of weeks. Turning or stirring it aerates it, which facilitates decomposition.

Yard and food waste make up more than 30% of the waste in our landfills. When you compost your kitchen and yard trimmings, you're helping to divert that waste from the landfill. It's a great way to live a more sustainable life.

For the last idea, we'll shift away from light and talk a bit about saving more water.

Self-Sustainability Idea #6 - How to Save More Water

It seems like half the country is dealing with a drought right now. Even if you're not in a drought, it makes good environmental sense to save as much water as possible. Now that doesn't mean you have to go without showering; your friends and family would probably not appreciate that degree of effort. However, there are other lifestyle changes and steps you can take to conserve water. And, you'll cut down on your water bill, too. Saving money is always good.

Step One: Install a Low Flow Shower Head

Low flow doesn't mean that your showers will be weak and unsatisfying. In fact, there are many powerful low flow showers that make you feel like you're in a spa. Older model showerheads generally have a flow rate of about five to eight gallons per minute. A low flow shower head uses about one and a half to two and a half gallons per minute. Simply unscrew your old model and attach the new model, then enjoy the savings.

Step Two: Xeriscape

Xeriscaping is the process of using plants in your landscaping that don't need much water. And we're not just talking about cacti and succulents. There's actually quite a large selection of plants that are drought friendly.

If xeriscaping isn't your style, consider watering your lawn in a more conservative manner. Water every couple of days, and water your lawn when the sun goes down. Water it for a solid twenty to thirty minutes to give it a good soaking. This helps the roots go deeper, and they'll be able to retrieve more water down deep, instead of relying on surface water.

Step Three: Laundry and Dishes

Only do complete loads of laundry and dishes. Don't run the appliances when they're less than full. The same is true when you're hand washing laundry or clothes. Fill the sink instead of letting the water run.

Every little step you can take to conserve water helps the environment. The changes don't have to be monumental to make a difference. Install a low flow toilet, take shorter showers, and pour any leftover water into plants. Be water wise!

The next sustainable living idea also embraces the resources that nature provides. Let's take a look at how to harvest your rainwater.

Self-Sustainability Idea #7 - Harvesting Rainwater

You don't have to be dealing with a drought to enjoy the sustainability benefits of harvesting rainwater. If you are in a drought, then you know that the hassle of alternating watering days can wreak havoc on your garden and landscaping.

Even if you're not in the midst of a drought, any rainwater harvesting system is a great way to reduce your water consumption. Rainwater harvesting reduces stress on local aquifers and rivers. When you reduce the stress, more water is available to help sustain aquatic life.

Step One: Review Your Home Codes and Laws

Make sure you can install a rainwater harvesting system. Some communities don't allow this, and some home organizations have strict guidelines on what your system can/cannot contain. Make sure you understand the rules; take them into consideration for the next step.

Step Two: Design Your System

The simplest system simply takes the rainwater from your downspout. You can buy rain barrels from your local home store, or you can create your own. If you only have room or a budget for one rain barrel, study your home's roofline and downspout system to identify the best place to collect water. You may find that one area of your roof gets the most flow. You'll gather the most water in this area.

Step Three: How Will You Use the Water?

It's important to create a system where you're using the rainwater. If it's allowed to sit, you'll start growing things and collecting bugs. In fact, it's a great place for mosquitos to reproduce.

You can attach a garden hose to your rain barrel and use it to water your garden. You can also create a drip irrigation system from your rain barrel. Or, you can simply fill watering cans from it and use the water to hydrate your plants both indoors and out.

Finally, take the time to occasionally clean out your rain barrel. Empty it completely and clean out the leaves and debris. You'll be amazed how much dirt and material can come off your roof, through your downspouts, and into your rain barrel. By cleaning it out, you'll ensure that the flow remains strong and that you don't start growing bacteria or fungus in your barrel.

Harvesting your rainwater is just one simple way you can take your sustainable lifestyle to the next level. You'll become more conscious of your water consumption. Don't be surprised if you never throw a glass of water down the drain ever again.

Make a Smooth Transition into Your New More Sustainable Lifestyle

There are so many ways to make a difference in the world and the environment. From composting, to installing a solar panel system in your home to provide your energy, there are so many options it might seem overwhelming. How do you decide where to even start, and more importantly - once you've decided, how do you make the transition a smooth one?

Step One: Prioritize and Plan

Choose one new habit, or one area of your life, where you want to make a change. What's the most important change you feel capable of tackling right now? Where do you think you can make the biggest difference? For example, maybe you want to start eating more organic and locally grown foods.

Once you've decided what's most important to you, consider how you can accomplish your goals. For example, if you want to eat more organic and locally grown foods you might join a CSA, add a garden to your yard, or visit the local farmer's market to get your produce.

This helps you add organic and locally grown produce to your daily life. It also helps cut down on emissions and your carbon footprint, because the food you're buying doesn't have to travel far to get to your table.

Step Two: Make Small Changes

Decide what you can do and take small steps. Your changes and goals should be realistic and achievable. For example, maybe gardening isn't really something you have time for, but you can visit the farmer's market once a week. That's a realistic goal that you can achieve.

Step Three: Be Patient and Persistent

Finally, keep in mind that it takes a few weeks to create a habit. Every step you take to live a more sustainable life is a positive step. Be patient with yourself and persistent in your life changes.

Chapter 18

Setting A Healthy Example

When you've taken all the right steps to intentionally change your body for the better, you'll be able to deal with the hurdles and set-backs with a much calmer mind. Target your expectations with a thorough plan and well-organized agenda to put your best foot forward, and, enjoy the process along the way. All your effort and enthusiasm will pay off in your own life, as well as affecting everyone you come in contact with. Loved ones, acquaintances, and casual contacts will be influenced by your dedication and genuine interest in taking care of yourself.

With a renewed perspective on health, and an obvious growth of knowledge, you will be someone that can offer guidance and compassion to others from your own experience. Being a good role model for those special people in your life can be motivation enough to stick with the battle of change. While you'll start out with many questions, possible frustrations, and an air of uncertainty, you can feel confident that will soon pass, and you can be one of the leaders of healthy living.

Through your individual choice to be healthier, whatever your underlying reasons are, you could be quite a committed example to many people around you. Hopefully, your positive example will rub off and start a chain reaction – a paradigm shift - to a better food supply and smarter generations that can alter the common thought that food is less important than it really is.

At one time in our human history, people could only source the 'natural' foods, as they are classified today. The hunter-gatherer diet of the past was completely plant-based with the addition of a meat product now and again. The body functions best when it's not overwhelmed with foreign substances that it's forced to process. Substances that are usable by the body, and are just waste products. The state of the filtering system of the human body is overused in the majority of cases. This constant strain from the numerous toxins entering the body through food, drink, and our environment, takes its toll in various ways through disease, discomfort, mental instability, and other physical impairments.

Be the change that many people want to see in the world. Change can be hard, but change for the better is so rewarding and self-gratifying that one can hardly help inspiring others to feel better, treat the environment better, and experience the paradigm shift that is slowly catching on throughout the world.

At this point, it's mainly just about you feeling good and getting your body in better shape. Your internal drive, planning and learning about a natural way to live, will keep you on track. Then, when you achieve some of your goals, you're going to, subconsciously, be impressing your new-found perspective on others.

The Future "PETRICK" Self-Sustainable Communities

An interviewer once asked me: "Dr. Petrick, how big is your vision?" I told her, I believe there has never been a better, more desperate time for a total revolution in this world. I am not talking about a government coup or revolt. There are no weapons needed or lives to be lost. Instead, I am talking about a revolution in healthcare, education, and how we build, live and thrive in our communities. We have the capability and engineering know-how to change the world by creating modernized self-sustainable communities - communities that give back, take less and beautify more.

Paradise, Indigo Bay, St. Maarten

One of my favorite examples of a self-sustainable community, and hopefully the community of the future, is the Indigo Bay project in St. Maarten, (on the Dutch side of the island). I had the pleasure to meet and interview the developers, Steve Smith and Mark Vandenburgh. These very ambitious, creative and forward-thinking men have taken an old world concept and added a modern twist.

Their masterpiece still in-creation is Indigo Bay, a magnificent 150-acre piece of pure, self-sustainable heaven. Indigo Bay has the most amazing white sand beaches, warm water, and the perfect tropical climate.

It is very obvious, when you drive around the property, that the developers were thinking many years into the future. They understand the needs and wants of the community and have plans to set aside grazing land for producing cattle (meat and milk), pork, chicken (meat and eggs), turkey; and they have already created three tilapia ponds.

Indigo Bay has plans for a large, commercial community garden that will produce vegetables for sale to the residents. The residents can either use the communal garden, or they have the option to be taught how to grow individual gardens in and/or around their homes. So basically, almost all of the food can be grown or raised right there inside the Indigo Bay community and sold back to the people. The vegetables, as well as the meat, will be pure and clean, with no pesticides, hormones or antibiotics.

Indigo Bay will utilize very large community windmills designed to create electricity to be used for the common areas in and around the community, like street lamps and electricity for the multi-purpose, non-denominational cultural center, the elementary school and the restaurants and shops that will be located inside the community. In addition, Indigo Bay also has plans for a micro-hydroelectric plant to harness the power from the rain that is plentiful in the islands.

There are full-scale plans for a fully-accredited medical school which will be attached to a hospital that is located inside the Indigo Bay community. They even planned for housing for the medical students that attend the college.

The "*HIP*" home designs are as modern as anything we have here in the United States, and the best part is that it is a self-sustainable community. The homes are built from local materials that are self-sustainable and natural materials to reduce costs and improve the living space. Each home will function somewhat like its own battery, with solar panels strategically positioned to maximize energy from the sun. The power produced can be used in the home, and the extra power can be sold back to the main grid that supports the neighboring communities, or it can be stored for emergencies and used inside Indigo Bay. It's a win-win for everybody. I truly believe that Indigo Bay could be the wave of the future for the next generation of communities, and I hope to help champion the self-sustainable movement.

About The Author

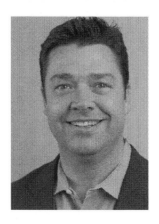

Dr. Jon S. Petrick is the clinical director of the Las Vegas Pain Relief Center. He specializes in Active Release Techniques, Stress Relief Method, Airway Restoration and other advanced chiropractic, functional therapies. For 10 years, he's been part of the Fox Sports Ultimate Fight Championship reality TV program. He has worked with several professional sports teams, including the major league Toronto Blue Jays minor league team the Las Vegas '51s. Currently, he works with hundreds of other professional athletes.

In addition, Dr. Petrick has worked for "Timet", a Nevada Corporation that produces Titanium. His work has saved Timet hundreds of thousands of dollars annually in reduced workers compensation costs. The hundreds of Timet employees celebrated over one million man hours without a worker's compensation claim recorded. He is the founder of Keep It Simple Make It Fun (KISMIF), an organization for individuals with mental and physical disabilities. He is currently working on a real-life documentary highlighting the benefits of Oxygen and Nitric Oxide therapy for Downs Syndrome children, athletes, veterans and other individuals with traumatic brain injuries.

To learn more about Dr. Jon, or how he can help you Get Off Your PATH and get on a path to a Self-Sustainable Lifestyle, or to attend one of his international seminars or lectures, visit with him directly at:

http://www.DrJonpetrick.com **or lasvegaspainreliefcenter.com**

Bonus Chapter

A Few Success Stories

There are typically four reasons people seek treatment from me:

1. Pain
2. Performance
3. Prevention
4. Self-sustaining lifestyle

I have over 20 years of experience helping thousands of athletes perfect their game or craft. Las Vegas Pain Relief Center (LVPRC) offers flexible scheduling to accommodate busy athletes and celebrities. We understand that today's professional athlete has very little time and often needs total privacy and professionalism. Since our highest priority is caring for our patients and athletes, here are a few examples of how we do that:

Anthony Pettis - Lightweight Champion

On a Wednesday evening in 2014, the phone rang at my Henderson, Nevada, office, and one of my staff members answered the phone. I immediately noticed that she had a sense of urgency on her face and tone in her voice. She said, "Dr. Petrick, there is an emergency phone call from a Dr. Jeffery Davidson, who is the head physician for the UFC (the Ultimate Fighting Championship). He has an urgent matter that he needs to discuss, and he said only with you."

I immediately grabbed the phone and said, "Hello, Dr. Davidson, this is Dr. Petrick. How can I help you sir?" He said, "Dr. Petrick. The UFC lightweight champion, Anthony Pettis, who is our Main pay-per-view event this Saturday night, has asked for you to see him. He has suffered a severe, right hip injury during his training camp and he is not sure if he can fight this weekend. We need you to examine, treat him and hopefully, fix him. We do not want to cancel the title fight. If we cancel, it will have a huge impact on this pay-per-view event and standings in the lightweight division."

So I told him to send Anthony over to my office, and I would see him immediately.

We waited only about a half hour for Anthony to make it to our office. I could tell, as soon as saw him, that he was in a great deal of pain and could not rotate properly on the hip. He could barely put any weight on the hip joint. I took him to my primary treatment and examination room. He indeed was in bad pain and needed the injury addressed or he would not be able to defend his title that Saturday. He had adhesions in his hip and some bruising. I performed a thorough examination and deemed his injury was strictly an injury to the soft tissues in the hip joint. The most likely cause of his hip injury was due to the soft tissue structures being damaged or sticking and binding together and not allowing tissue sliding to occur between the belly of the muscles or tendons. In a sense, his hip was being jammed up and pinching the hip joint. I treated him with Active Release Techniques on the damaged tissues, which helped address the fascia adhesions in and around the hip joint. I used the Stress Relief Method to make sure he was not in the twist, and I also manipulated his hip joint and made sure it was articulating properly. Once we finished with the hour long treatment, we needed to put the treatment to the test and see if he would be able to use the hip without pain.

I escorted Anthony to the gymnasium to have him try out the hip. He tried to roundhouse kick the heavy bag several times, to see if the kicking motion would reproduce the hip pain. He kicked the bag about 15 to 20 times and could not duplicate or reproduce the pain. He was grateful and very happy he had no pain, but more importantly, he would be able to fight and defend his title.

I phoned Dr. Davidson and advised him that "THE FIGHT IS ON." Dr. Davidson was very excited to know that the emergency had passed and that Anthony would be ready to fight on Saturday.

FIGHT NIGHT…. I was obviously watching the fight… after all, it was my work on the line, and I needed to make sure everything went well. Cut to the chase, Anthony successfully defended his title in a lopsided victory over Gilbert Melendez, To make it even better, he landed several of the hardest roundhouse kicks that he has ever thrown and the hip was unaffected.

This is just one example of how my care works on high profile acute cases, with all the stress a doctor could ask for. It felt good to know that we helped a top level athlete defend his title, not to mention I felt great to be the sole person to make a pay-per view event happen.

Jay Cutler - 4 time Mr. Olympia

I received a phone call in my office from a gentleman who, at the time, was making a comeback on the professional bodybuilder's circuit. His name was Mr. Jay Cutler. He was a four-time Mr. Olympia and ranked as one of the top bodybuilders in the entire world, but unfortunately, he suffered a few serious injuries that had kept him on the sideline and out of competition, or at least the podium. He was calling me because he was excited to do something no one has ever done, and that was win a Mr. Olympia at 40 years old.

His injuries were almost as great as his size at over 300 lbs. He had a left shoulder problem associated with a torn bicipital ligament, as well as a right-sided hamstring tear, or issue, near the top of the hamstring attachment in the hip. This is important as there are not too many people who know how to successfully treat these types of injuries in these areas. The tissues were starting to fray and pull apart from the actual bony attachment, so needless to say, I had my work cut out for me. It was going to be an uphill battle to get him to that top level again. But nobody knows their body like big Jay.

It takes years and years of dedication and determination to become the best in the world at any sport, and when you're dealing with athletes who expect perfection, it can be a little stressful.

I told him to come into the office and I would meet him there. I would do a thorough examination and treat his injuries. After we met and I examined him, it did not take me long to find out where the adhesions were in the tissue(s) and utilized the Active Release Techniques to increase the sliding motion in and around the muscles and tendons. There was an immediate improvement to the Adductor Magnus, or inside of the hamstring, and an immediate increase in strength and range of motion in the torn left bicep. The bicep was preventing him from getting a full workout, as he did not have full range of motion, which prohibited him from getting his left arm underneath a squat bar, or doing a full bench or biceps work out.

After the first session or treatment and the success we had, we continued to treat Jay approximately 2 to 3 times a week for about 6 weeks leading up to the Mr. Olympia.

Although Jay originally had come to me for pain, it was also for prevention and performance. Of course he wanted to perform without pain, but he also wanted to perform at his very best and prevent injuries from occurring in the first place.

For me, there is absolutely nothing more gratifying then when I can help an athlete, as finely tuned and as perfectly constructed as Jay

Cutler, and I can make him even better. Wow, what a rush that is! Then to keep them at that top level and out of pain is amazing.

This is another example of how my care not only works for acute or chronic conditions, but also how I am called upon and utilized for pain relief, prevention and performance.

William Walters - Entrepreneur

Another one of my success stories has to do with a gentleman by the name of William Walters. 60 Minutes actually did a story on him, because he's one of the world's biggest gamblers. He helps set the tone for the gambling lines for Las Vegas and he owns several golf courses, car dealerships, and other major business ventures. He was having a really bad problem with his foot, and his golf game was shot. He had come to me through a referral, and I had done such a good job of treating his problem that he decided that he needed the treatment every day until the problem was resolved. The only problem was that he lived in Carlsbad, California, and he needed to be there, and I needed to be here. He was so grateful that I was able to help him that he asked me if he could fly me down. He asked, "What would it take for me to fly you down to Carlsbad so that you can treat myself, my wife, and my staff?" So, he flew me down on his corporate jet, and as he said "I worked my magic." To this day he continues to recommend me, and still flies me down on occasion to Carlsbad for me to work on him and his entire staff. I've made not only a life-long patient, but also a good friend.

Ian Naismith

I had the privilege and honor of meeting a fine gentleman by the name of Ian Naismith. It was kind of like "a small world" type of connection. Besides once being a heavyweight professional boxer, his grandfather,

James Naismith, invented the game of basketball in Laurence, Kansas, in 1891.

Ian was wanting to make sure the Naismith name stayed true, pure and honorable; so he ended up in this legal battle for the actual rules as written. He ended up obtaining and owning the rules to basketball, the actual documents themselves. He would go around the country doing interviews, trying to bring these fundamental sporting rules back, so they started calling him 'The Basketball Man.'

It was right around a year later a very close friend called me and told me that Ian had suffered a horrible stroke. The stroke ultimately left him paralyzed, and the doctors were telling him he wasn't going to get any better. He was in bad shape, and for over 12 months he remained in poor condition. But once he was able to walk and talk a little, I talked him into coming to Las Vegas and seeing what we could do to get him back on his feet.

I was dealing with the worst of the worst, if you will, and I didn't know what was going to happen. There were times, when we were working with him, where he went to the doctor's office and they would try to deflate his optimism and drive, but they were not successful. They released him and he came to me. I noticed that he was not breathing right, so I said," IAN, let me listen to your lungs and take some x-rays." Sure enough, he had pneumonia. If I hadn't take those x-rays, he would have died. That was all the trust he needed in me, because I found something by listening and being a good doctor. He just wasn't feeling right, and we knew something was up. Over the next few months, we treated him and gave him a new lease on life in his late 60's. We got him on the right diet. We got him doing exercises, mainly curls. I'm not kidding when I tell you that in the last few years of his life, he could do 1,000 curls. He could do it with both arms. It wasn't 100 lbs., but with small weights of 25 to 30 lbs. He was obsessive with it. He was just constantly wanting to do better. His mindset changed - he didn't want to be an old man. He wanted to fight to be better. He wanted to be a young man, and it was like we got him doing different things and feeling better. I got him better shoes so he wasn't at risk of falling due to shoes that weren't really good for him.

Due to all the work we did with him, he had a resurgence of life. He was able to drive around the country, after all of this, and promote his movie and story of the "The Basketball Man." He helped assure the Naismith name was synonymous with a gentleman's sport, like it was created to be and how it should be. Because of the work that we had done, he was able to present the first sportsmanship award to the national basketball star, Steve Nash. The **NBA Sportsmanship Award** is now an annual National Basketball Association (NBA) award given to a player who most "exemplifies the ideals of sportsmanship on the court with ethical behavior, fair play, and integrity."

He ended up living a really great life. Part of that had to do with some of the mental mapping that we had done when we visited him in North and South Carolina.

Throughout the years, he had credited me in helping him get his body back. Unfortunately, while on a train to see me for treatment (because he refused to fly), he peacefully passed away at the age of 73.

Special Offer

I have established the lowest possible pricing for all of the items in this book that are needed to become self-sustainable. If you are interested in any or all of the products that you find in this book, simply go to my website at **Getoffyourpath.com** and you will be able to get substantial discounts, guaranteed.

Tools needed for the Self-Sustainable Lifestyle

- **Foam roll**
- **Cook bands**
- **Kettle bells (3 sizes)**
- **Heart-rate monitor**
- **Home weight scale**
- **Food scale**
- **Water body**
- **Products (powders and pills)**
- **Yoga mat**
- **Towels**
- **Journal**
- **Medicine ball**

Off the Grid Equipment

- **Intellibed Mattress**
- **Tower garden**
- **Solar Panels**
- **Windmill**
- **Water Harvesting equipment**
- **Composting unit**
- **Personal Use Hyperbaric chamber**